Fingernail Biting

Fingernail Biting

Theory, Research and Treatment

Norman H. Hadley, Ph.D.

Associate Professor
Department of Educational Psychology
Memorial University of Newfoundland
St. John's, Newfoundland

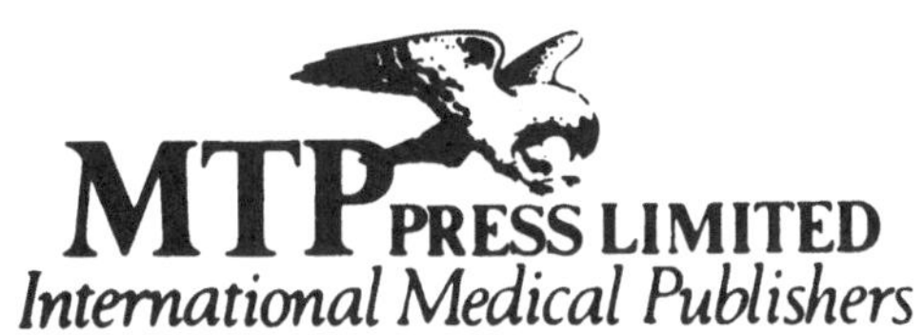

ISBN-13:978-94-011-6325-5 e-ISBN-13:978-94-011-6323-1
DOI: 10.1007/978-94-011-6323-1

Softcover reprint of the hardcover 1st edition 1984

Published in the UK and Europe by
MTP Press Limited
Falcon House
Lancaster, England

Published in the US by
SPECTRUM PUBLICATIONS, INC.
175-20 Wexford Terrace
Jamaica, NY 11432

Foreword

Everyone exhibits styles of movement and speech, traits and habits which are characteristic of them as people but do not contribute directly to their purposeful activity at any one time. Many of these will be expressions of personality of which the individual may be unaware or even cherish and which evoke a favorable or neutral response from others. Conversely, displays such as gross involuntary tics or compulsive rituals are a burden to the sufferer and are socially embarrassing or obnoxious. These may be manifestations of a more fundamental neurotic disorder or the product of deep-seated maladaptive learning. Nail-biting occupies a central position along such a spectrum. Although it may serve as a tension-reducing or other functional device, few nail-biters would not wish to be rid of the habit but find it as difficult to eliminate as, say, an addiction to smoking. Even so, it cannot be considered abnormal in a psychiatric sense in that many nail-biters exhibit none of the traits and symptoms characteristic of mental disorder.

Various explanations from varying theoretical standpoints have been proposed to account for the development and persistence of nail-biting and even more strategies have been suggested for its control. A dispassionate review of the extensive but scattered literature is very welcome and I can think of no-one better equipped to provide that review than Dr. Hadley. I first met Dr. Hadley several years ago, when he came to my Department at the University of Leeds as a graduate student to carry out original research in this very area. He proved to be a most conscientious and enterprising investigator and an indefatigable scholar. This book is not intended for the presentation of his own valuable empirical findings but brings together all the view-points and findings on the nature, correlates, assessment and treatment of nail-biting of the past half-century. This historical perspective discloses a marked trend away from more speculative clinical accounts to behaviorally based empirical investigations. The latter provide promising leads for the development of effective self-management techniques for control of the habit. Thus, although the book is intended for clinicians and researchers, it will also be of considerable interest to many nail-biters.

H. GWYNNE JONES
Emeritus Professor
University of Leeds
Senior Research Fellow
University of Birmingham
United Kingdom

Preface

The preparation of this volume has entailed a thorough study of the nailbiting literature beginning with the studies of the 1930s. The coverage of the journal articles and other sources of information over five decades has provided a historical perspective on the topic of nailbiting. The literature revealed a definite shift in emphasis from early psychodynamic formulations to the contemporary trend toward empirical investigations and a focus on awareness and self-controlling responses in the management of nailbiting behavior.

Chapter 1 discusses the significance of nailbiting as an undesirable response and the various ways it is classified in the medical and psychological literature.

Chapter 2 explains various measurement techniques for assessing fingernail growth. It describes techniques that can be conveniently used during therapy for fingernail biting as well as various procedures that are used in pure research studies designed to investigate aspects of nail growth. Chapter 3 discusses the relationship between nailbiting and personality characteristics, familial variables, intelligence, specific situational factors, and other behavioral problems. Part of the chapter examines age and sex trends associated with nailbiting.

Chapter 4 presents and discusses in detail different theoretical formulations about the etiology of nailbiting.

In Chapter 5, the focus is on various types of behavioral intervention. Specific remedial approaches are discussed within the context of a number of representative published research studies. Sufficient detail is provided to give the clinician an appreciation of the advantages and potential problems associated with each technique.

It is difficult to draw specific conclusions about the causes of fingernail biting or to single out one treatment procedure as being most effective, because one cannot generalize about these issues. Nailbiting seems to be an individual problem to which a number of theories and treatment strategies could apply, depending on factors such as the severity of the nailbiting, the situations associated with the nailbiting, and the individual's history of the problem. All of these factors must be considered in designing an effective remedial strategy.

I hope that the mental health researcher and clinician will find this book useful.

CONCLUDING STATEMENT

The significance of this monograph is twofold. First, it provides information on the basis of which testable hypotheses can be developed. Second, it is obvious from this review of the nailbiting literature that a number of complex biological, psychological, and sociological variables must be considered in attempting to understand an individual's nailbiting behavior. Consequently, the designing of effective methods for nailbiting prevention and treatment would be facilitated by a multidimensional model of nailbiting.

Norman H. Hadley

Acknowledgments

I would like to express my thanks to the researchers who responded to my personal communications in a helpful and encouraging way. I am especially indebted to the following individuals who provided detailed comments and suggestions: Dr. B. D. Bucher, Dr. V. J. Adesso, Dr. R. S. Jones, Dr. H. H. Work, and Dr. C. Fanta. A special word of thanks goes to Professor H. Gwynne Jones for writing the foreword to the book.

I also want to express my gratitude to Maurice Ancharoff, President of SP Medical and Scientific Books, Inc. With good-humored patience, sensible advice and painstaking care, he provided the guidance necessary to bring the work to fruition. Isabel Stein is certainly deserving of my thanks and appreciation for her very careful and thorough editorial work on my manuscript.

Words are extremely inadequate to express my deep and sincere feelings of gratitude to my wife, Paula. I thank her for the many long hours she spent in helping me with library research and with the endless number of revisions to almost every paragraph of the book. Her ability to organize ideas and synthesize information helped me to complete the manuscript long before I would have on my own. In spite of me neglecting many personal obligations to her, she unselfishly gave her help, emotional support, and encouragement throughout the entire two-year project.

Contents

1

Significance and Medical Classification of Nailbiting

A careful study of the nailbiting literature has revealed the need for a thorough review that encompasses and systematically presents the theoretical considerations and treatment formulations of a number of researchers. To date, no such compendium is available. Early theorists presented their views on the etiology of nailbiting primarily within a psychodynamic framework and often without an empirical data base. In contrast, many published reports of contemporary empirical investigations dealing with the treatment of nailbiting behavior lack a theoretically based discussion. This, however, may be due to the difficulty in translating the early theoretical models into therapeutic procedures. This monograph is an attempt to delineate a number of salient issues pertinent to the study of nailbiting, to clearly describe and synthesize the theories that have been presented to date in the literature, and to discuss various treatments for nailbiting.

EMOTIONAL SIGNIFICANCE OF NAILBITING

Reference was made to the significance of the nailbiting problem by Stephen and Koenig (1970), who stated: "Many young adults define severe nail-biting as a significant problem for them in terms of both physical discomfort and as a socially offensive trait" (p. 211).

Azrin and Nunn (1977) examined and described the special importance of fingernail biting behavior from the perspective of the individual. The seriousness of the problem was demonstrated by the following typical statements made by nailbiters:

> "I die of shame when I'm typing at work and someone stares at my hands."
>
> "When anyone is around, I keep my fingers folded into my palm to hide my nails."
>
> "I love to play cards, but I don't dare."
>
> "Other girls make their nails look beautiful with all kinds of nail polish, but when I tried it once, it only attracted attention to their ugliness."
>
> "If a coin or small object falls on the floor, I feel as if I'm wearing mittens, it's so hard to pick it up."
>
> "It looks ugly when I gnaw my nails, I'm sure, because it looks ugly to me when I see others doing it."
>
> "I've given up on using Scotch tape. I can't get at the edge of the tape no matter what I do."
>
> "I sometimes wonder how my boyfriend can enjoy holding my hand."
>
> "My friends laugh at me. And my parents, nag, nag, nag!"
>
> "It's bad enough that I do it, but now my kids are starting to do it too."
>
> "When I'm alone driving in my car, that's when I nibble away the most."
>
> "I cringe when I see my hands in the mirror. What other people must think when they look at my stubby fingers!" [Azrin and Nunn, 1977, pp. 9-10]

Pennington and Mearin emphasized that nailbiting "will always remain the problem of the individual case" (1944, p. 630). In a study involving 533 naval recruits who were nailbiters, Pennington and Mearin concluded that the significance of nailbiting "is best revealed by each recruit's reaction to his own hands and to the questions of the examiner" (p. 630). Pennington and Mearin found that the recruit who faces the fact that he bites his nails and who recognizes that he should break his habit is not as likely to have other nervous symptoms that are psychiatrically disqualifying for military service as is the one who denies that he is a nailbiter or the recruit who admits that he bites when worried or emotionally disturbed. Of the 46 nailbiters who indicated that they bit their nails most when upset, 39% were required to undergo further psychiatric examination. The 32 who denied that they bit their fingernails had a 21% holdover rate. These two groups represented the largest percentages of those who underwent further psychiatric assessment.

According to Illingworth, nailbiting is a harmless habit, though it looks unpleasant and spoils the nails. He cautioned, however:

> The danger of the habit lies more in the attitude of the parents. Excessive efforts to stop it can cause quite a lot of unpleasantness and are much more likely to fix the habit and cause its continuation than to stop it. . . . In some children it becomes an attention-seeking device, and continues because of determined efforts to stop it. [Illingworth, 1964, p. 51]

In their booklet, *Nailbiting and Cuticlebiting: Kicking the Habit*, Perkins and Perkins (1976) stressed that nailbiting is a useless habit that does not enhance the appearance of the hands. The individual also runs the risk of having his nailbiting behavior mistakenly interpreted as an "inner problem." Perkins and Perkins argued that:

> Nailbiting is more than useless, it is damaging. The view that nailbiting is a symptom of a more deepseated problem has its roots in older schools of psychology and although it is no longer believed by many professionals, this misconception is still widely held among lay people. The unfortunate nailbiter must therefore contend with the armchair interpretations of amateur Freuds who interpret gnawed nails as evidence of inner turmoil. [Perkins and Perkins, 1976, p. 1]

The results of a survey of children's behavioral problems by Rutter (1967) indicated that nailbiting among children may not be symptomatic of psychopathology. The purpose of the survey was to assess the validity of a children's behavioral questionnaire designed by Rutter for completion by teachers. In attempting to do this, Rutter compared nonclinic schoolchildren with children attending a psychiatric clinic. The results that pertained to the nailbiting item (Item 13, "Frequently bites nails or fingers") are presented in Table 1, which is adapted from a more detailed summary of the data in the Rutter study. It indicates the number and percentage of children in the neurotic, antisocial, and control groups who scored 1, denoting "certainly applies," or 2, indicating "applies somewhat" on the nailbiting item (Rutter, 1967). The teachers' ratings indicated that the percentage of children who bit their nails was approximately the same in the normal, neurotic, and antisocial groups. Nailbiting was not included in the list of items that "discriminate between the groups at a significance level of 5 per cent or better" (Rutter, 1967, p. 6).

In the third edition of *The Technique of Psychotherapy*, Wolberg (1977) viewed nailbiting as a "common outlet for tension in preadolescence and adolescence" and acknowledged that "it may persist as a neurotic symptom into adult life" (p. 1,025). Wolberg added: "They [nailbiters] are usually unaware that the nailbiting symptom has a meaning, and they are often puzzled by the persistence of the urge to chew their finger tips" (p. 934).

Sim and Finn regarded the nailbiting habit as "a normal tension release," even though parents may not consider it to be "socially acceptable" (1973, p. 380). They noted that nailbiting is generally not indicative of psychopathology: "A normal habit . . . [such as] nail biting . . . should not be considered bad unless it does actual harm either physically or morally to the child himself or to others about him. Nail biting generally does neither" (1973, p. 380).

Rarely is a child brought to a physician because of fingernail biting. In most instances, the physician discovers incidentally, through inquiry or inspection, that the nails are being bitten. Kanner described nailbiting as "the most widespread of all forms of habitual manipulations of the body" (1972, p. 528). Although he said it may indicate some personality difficulty, he cautioned that we "cannot consider it as 'an exquisitely psychopathic symptom' " (p. 528). The findings of Ballinger indicated that "nail-biting is not an important psychiatric symptom" (1970, p. 446), a conclusion based on the fact that his study revealed no significant differences in the prevalence of nailbiting among mentally ill, mentally retarded, and normal populations in England. Prevalence in the psychiatric group appeared to be related to age rather than to mental illness.

Table 1 Children Scoring 1 or 2 on the Nailbiting Item of Rutter's Behavioral Questionnaire

Item	*Antisocial boys*		*Antisocial girls*		*Neurotic boys*		*Neurotic girls*		*Control boys*		*Control girls*	
No.	*No.*	*Percent*	*No.*	*Percent*	*No.*	*Percent*	*No.*	*Percent*	*No.*	*Percent*	*No.*	*Percent*
13	11	17.46	14	35.00	5	16.67	7	22.58	39	25.16	32	24.43
Total	63		40		30		31		155		131	

Adapted from "A Children's Behaviour Questionnaire for Completion by Teachers: Preliminary Findings," by M. Rutter, *Journal of Child Psychology and Psychiatry*, 1967, *8*, 1-11. Copyright by the Association of Child Psychology and Psychiatry and reprinted with permission.

The attitude toward nailbiting in the early 1950s was to "recognize nail biting as a distress signal" (Rushforth, 1951, p. 193). According to Rushforth, nailbiting was associated with anxiety, the causes of which could be determined by monitoring the activities of the child and noting the situations during which the child bites his nails. She wrote that "observant parents will report that the habit fluctuates, and if they are asked to watch the conditions under which it becomes active it may give them increasing insight into the causes of their child's anxiety" (Rushforth, p. 193). The "distress signal" function of nailbiting was also applied to adult nailbiters, in whom it might "accompany the early development of hyperthyroid activity of nervous origin or other psychosomatic illness" (Rushforth, p. 194). Rushforth claimed that in anxiety cases the nailbiting mannerism "is compulsive but under a degree of control" (p. 192). She based this view on the reports of women who indicated that although they were unable to stop nailbiting, they did not bite so much as to entirely ruin the look of their hands.

Shahovitch (1945) introduced her discussion of nailbiting by emphasizing that an infantile pattern of nailbiting is often evident among kindergarten children. Frequently, the child puts his hand to his mouth and sucks one of his fingers. This may cause softening and possible breaking of the fingernail, which is subsequently bitten as the child goes to sleep. This is not the pattern followed by the true nailbiter, however, who is "beginning to partake of the problems of adult life" (Shahovitch, p. 302). The real nailbiting problem, according to Shahovitch, begins in the first grade among children who feel timid and uncertain in making the transition from kindergarten to the first grade at school. The problem generally dissipates by the age of 12, however, after which very few children acquire the habit.

Whereas data are available on the behavioral problems of children who have been referred to child guidance clinics, few reports of the behavioral problems of a cross-section of normal children have been published. Macfarlane, Allen, and Honzik (1954), however, have provided a detailed account of the behavioral problems of a group of 126 normal children who comprised the control group in their longitudinal California guidance study. The children in both the control group and the Guidance Group constituted a representative sample of the children in the much larger Berkeley Survey, which included every third child born in Berkeley between January 1, 1928, and June 30, 1929. Physical examinations and mental tests were given to the control group (normal) children at regular intervals. The larger portion of the data, however, were obtained from the mothers whenever they brought their children to the clinic for testing. The infrequency of these visits and the fact that as the children grew older, the mothers did not always accompany the children, presented some difficulties to the data-collecting program for the control children. The moving away of families from the area or loss of interest and subsequent withdrawal from the study also created some problems in data collecting. When the children were 21 months old, reports were made by the mothers of 116 of the 126 children in the control group. A gradual decline in the number of reports occurred, and when the children were 14 years of age, only 41 mothers' reports were given.

For purposes of data collection, specific behavior and personality codes ranging from 1 to 5 were devised to represent answers to questions on the recording form. With regard to the nailbiting item, i.e., "Does he bite his nails [?]" (Macfarlane et al., 1954, p. 64), the following categories of answers were provided:

> (1) Extreme and persistent biting of nails or cuticle around nails. Bitten "down to the quick"; fingers disfigured.
> (2) Nails kept chewed down [less severe than (1)] but fingers not disfigured.
> (3) Mild persistent biting of nails; always evidence of chewed nails.
> (4) Mild periodic biting of nails, or pulling of rough nails.
> (5) Never bites nails; if nails are broken or rough, uses file or scissors or asks mother to. [p. 25]

Categories 1 through 4 indicated descriptions that were coded as problems. Hence, only the behavioral description "never bites nails" was considered to be nonproblematic. Over half of the children in the study were assigned to Category 5, which led the authors to conclude the nailbiting was a good example of a behavior that was not normally distributed.

From a statistical viewpoint, nailbiting may not be considered a significant problem for "normal" children, as indicated by the results of the Macfarlane et al. study. Statistics do not, however, reflect the significance of the problem to the individual, either in terms of the discomfort or embarrassment it may cause or in terms of its potential for contributing to other problems, for example, those related to dentition.

NAILBITING AND DENTITION

Kerr, Ash, and Millard stressed that fingernail biting is "of importance in dentistry because of its association with malocclusion, trauma to teeth, and gingivitis" (1978, p. 112). The significance of nailbiting as a potential factor contributing to problems in dentition is evident in their three-point discussion:

> [1] In the presence of diseases of the nails such as onychomycosis and mycotic paronchyia, nail biting may spread the causative agent of the nail disease to the mouth. . . . [(2) Chronic nailbiting should be correlated] with small fractures of the incisal edges of the anterior teeth and with gingivitis associated with the trauma from continual nail biting; [(3)] It is necessary that the nail biting habit be eliminated before satisfactory periodontal therapy or restorative therapy can be undertaken. [Kerr et al., 1978, pp. 112-113]

Ackerman and Proffit (1975) also identified nailbiting as one of the common childhood habits that affect dentition. Corn and Marks have indicated that "thumb sucking followed by nail biting can initiate orofacial muscle dysfunction" (1976, p. 275).

Geiger and Hirschfeld (1974), in a text dealing with malocclusion of teeth in children, recommended that as part of the diagnosis, a child's fingernails and cuticles should be examined. Their rationale was that constant fingernail biting may result in malpositioning of the teeth. Geiger and Hirschfeld considered nailbiting to be one of the habits that "transmit the entire force of the musculature from a tooth through the intermediate object to the opposing tooth" (1974, p. 63). In the text *Applied Psychology in Dentistry*, Manhold (1972) included nailbiting in a list of habits that contribute to periodontal disease.

Sim and Finn argued that nailbiting is not a harmful habit that produces malocclusion because "the forces or stresses applied in nail biting are similar to those in the chewing process" (1973, p. 380).

They acknowledged, however, that persistent nailbiting may lead to "a marked attrition of the lower anterior teeth" (p. 380) if grit is present under the nails during nailbiting episodes. Moyers noted that "nail-biting is mentioned frequently as a cause of tooth malpositions," but in describing the relation of nailbiting to dentition he claimed that "the malocclusion associated with this habit [nailbiting] is likely to be of a . . . localized nature" (1973, p. 259).

From a review of a number of surveys of nailbiting prevalence, Massler and Malone (1950) concluded that:

> Nailbiting is "normal" in children from 4 years of age until adolescence, in the sense that "normal" indicates averageness or the commonplace. On the other hand, the low prevalence rate after 18 years of age may indicate that nailbiting, except the very mildest kind, should be considered "abnormal." Certainly after the age of 30, nailbiting should be considered more seriously than merely as a habit. [p. 524]

Massler and Malone offered the interpretation that "nailbiting . . . may be normal or abnormal, desirable or undesirable, depending upon the conditions under which it occurs" (p. 528). They recommended that nailbiting be assessed in the light of the interplay of four specific conditions: "(1) the age of the nailbiter, (2) intensity and frequency of the action, (3) relation to the situation in which it occurs, and (4) the emotional status of the biter" (Massler and Malone, p. 528).

MEDICAL CLASSIFICATION OF NAILBITING

Diversity is evident in the classification of nailbiting. Although there is some consensus of agreement in the literature, nailbiting behavior has been included in a variety of categories. It has been termed a behavior disorder, secondary habit disturbance, personality disorder, tic, problem associated with motor manifestations, self-stimulating behavior, and a habitual body movement.

Anthony included nailbiting in his discussion of "what [behaviors] should or should not be regarded as abnormal" (1970, p. 668). Generally, a problem behavior such as nailbiting was "regarded as a symptom rather than as an entity" (Anthony, 1970, p. 668) and could be differentiated from normal behavior on the basis of its greater intensity, frequency, and persistence. Azrin and Nunn indicated similar criteria, as reflected in their statement, "the great persistence or high frequency of the mannerism is what makes it a problem" (1977, p. 33). In these instances of greater intensity, frequency, and persistence, the behavior is more likely to be expressed "by both patient and clinician as 'different' . . . more likely to be associated with other symptoms and to be embedded in an overtly pathogenic environment" (Anthony, 1970, p. 668).

Anthony compiled a brief historical review of the various interpretations of nailbiting behavior. The following trends were noted:

> Kanner (1960) offered a capsular history of nail biting from the literature over a period of 25 years. In 1908, nail biting was regarded as "a stigma of degeneration"; in 1912 it was seen as "an exquisite psychopathic symptom"; and in 1931 it was described as "a sign of an unresolved Oedipus complex." Following this, a survey indicated that 66% of school children had been nail-biters at some time or another, which led Kanner to remark that it was "hardly realistic to assume that two-thirds of our youth are degenerate, exquisitely psychopathic or walking around with an unresolved Oedipus complex." [Anthony, 1970, p. 668]

Nailbiting is among the behaviors discussed in the context of "secondary habit disturbances" by Maddison, Day, and Leadbeater (1975). In their psychiatric nursing text, they defined a habit disturbance in children as a type of adjustment reaction to stress. They distinguished between two main types of habit disturbances. The so-called primary habit disturbances relate to "those functions that normally develop a habitual pattern at a fairly early age, in particular eating, sleeping and excretion" (p. 285). The specific disturbances included in this classification were feeding disorders, disturbances in sleeping habits, enuresis, and encopresis. According to Maddison et al., secondary habit disturbances "represent more than a simple failure to establish the habit patterns of the normal child" (p. 286). Thumb-sucking was included in the category of secondary habit disturbances under the classification of "gratification habits"–those that are pleasurable to the child. Nailbiting, on the other hand, was classified as a tension habit, i.e., as a habit "seen in the tense child who is directing his aggression towards himself" (Maddison et al., p. 287).

In another psychiatric nursing text, nailbiting was discussed in the context of "habit and conduct disorders" (Gibson, 1971, p. 121). According to Gibson, nailbiting "is common and occasionally persists into adult life . . . it occurs in children who are unhappy or worried" (p. 121). With regard to the informal diagnosis of children's behavior disorders, Fremont, Seifert, and Wilson (1977) suggested that nailbiting is a possible symptom of conduct and personality disorder; problems such as nailbiting, which are frequently displayed by children in the classroom, should be "targets of concern" (Fremont et al., p. 20).

Redl and Wattenberg (1959) described nailbiting as belonging "to the family of *oral habits*, like thumb sucking, pencil chewing, gum chewing, and pipe smoking" (p. 54).

The motoric aspect of the nailbiting mannerism has been considered by some researchers. Macfarlane et al. (1954), for example, included nailbiting in their list of "Problems Associated with Motor Manifestations" (p. 12). Shaw and Lucas (1970) asserted that some authorities (unspecified) classify nailbiting as a tic, but they questioned this for at least two reasons: (a) a true tic is "spasmodic, sudden, and involuntary" (p. 357), whereas nailbiting is more readily controlled; (b) nailbiting frequently occurs before age six, while this is rarely the case with true tics.

Although not very common, there is a fingernail-associated motor mannerism, which is classified as a "habit-tic deformity" by Samman (1972). It is mentioned in this discussion because persistent playing with the nails is considered by several writers to be related to nailbiting (Azrin and Nunn, 1977; Bucher, 1968). In describing the nail manipulation, Samman (1972) wrote:

> The deformity usually consists of a depression down the centre of one nail with numerous horizontal ridges extending across the nail from it. The depression is sometimes missing. The deformity is usually confined to one or both thumb-nails and is caused by the patient picking at the cuticle . . . or stroking the nail of the affected digit with a finger of the same hand. [p. 1660]

The typical deformity produced by this mannerism is illustrated in Figure 1. Honigman (1975) also considered "mechanical manipulation of the nail . . . by a finger or device" as a habit-tic, which could result in "various deformities and even loss of the nail" (p. 1556).

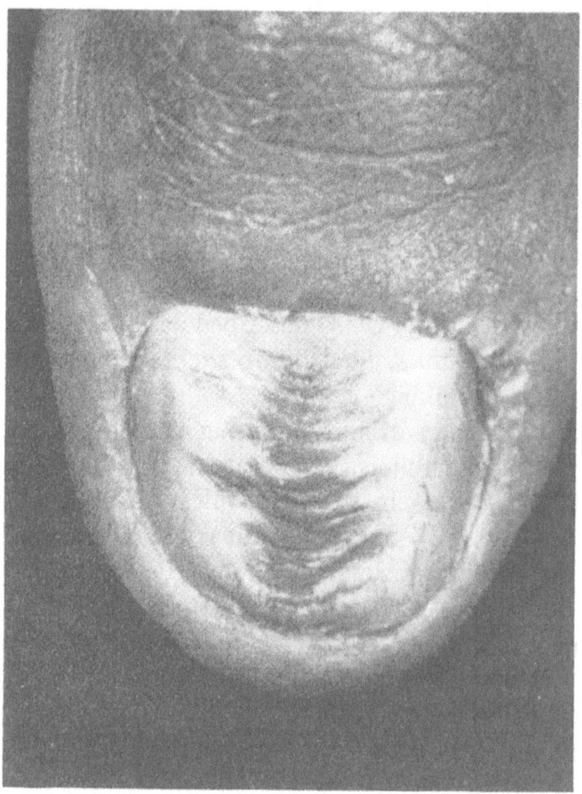

Figure 1 Deformity caused by playing with nails (habit tic). St. John's Hospital. From "The Nails," by P. D. Samman, in A. Rook, D. S. Wilkinson, and F. J. G. Ebling (eds.), *Textbook of dermatology* (2d ed., vol. 2). London: Blackwell, 1972, p. 1660. Copyright by Blackwell Scientific Publishers Ltd.; reprinted with permission.

Slater and Roth (1969) classified nailbiting as a habitual body movement and argued that nailbiting is not synonymous with a tic:

> [Nailbiting] and other *habitual manipulations* of certain parts of the body can, however, be distinguished from tics. They have not the sudden onset and short time-pattern of the tic; unlike tics they are not repeated in the photographically identical form; and they are more obviously purposive in providing pleasure. Subjectively they are felt to be under volitional control, and

they always involve two parts of the body at the same time, one of which is usually the hand. [p. 655]

Blair, Jones, and Simpson (1975), in an educational psychology text, included fingernail biting in their list of symptoms that "may point to handicaps and learning difficulties"; nailbiting was considered a "type of defect" signifying "emotional disturbances" (p. 337). Jones cautioned, however, that "any one symptom such as nailbiting taken in isolation should not be given undue weight in calling a child (or adult) emotionally disturbed" (Jones, personal communication). He added that many individuals "have personal 'nervous habits' " and that "perhaps most significant is the *increase* of such behavior[s] under stress."

Sarles and Heisler (1978) classified nailbiting as a self-stimulating behavior rather than as a symptom of psychopathology. In their words: "[Nailbiting does] not generally signify psychological maladjustment and thus often require[s] little intervention other than reassurance for the parents and the recommendation for adequate stimulation of the child" (p. 590).

Mitchell (1973) classified fingernail biting as a habit disorder, a category of behavior disorders that involved habitual manipulations of various parts of the body. He indicated that a habit disorder such as nailbiting could be distinguished from a tic in the following ways: "[Nailbiting is] carried out at a higher level of consciousness, may be performed continuously for long periods, can be interrupted, [is] under voluntary control, and [is] usually pleasurable" (p. 389). Nailbiting was also listed as a habit disorder by Stone (1976), who believed that "nail-biting . . . [is not] harmful or ominous in itself, but if it provokes constant and excessively anxious responses from parents this can be the starting-point for 'relationship disorders' " (p. 81).

Only recently has attention been drawn to the revision of psychiatric classification systems so as to include the behavioral problems of children and youth. Jenkins stated that the American Psychiatric Association's *Diagnostic and Statistical Manual of Mental Disorders* (DSM-I) made primarily two distinctions in its classification of behavior disorders: those that are "caused by or associated with impairment of brain tissue function and those which are not" (Jenkins, 1973, p. 21). This classification, however, had little to offer in the way of classifying the behavioral problems of children and youth.

Jenkins further suggested that the course usually followed was to classify many children's disorders as "transient situational disorders" (p. 22). The problem with this category was that:

> With the persistence of external pressure and resultant maladaptive response, the pattern of the maladaptive response gradually becomes more and more ingrained, more and more internalized. Most of the problems we see in children *begin* as situational reactions. That is to say, in most psychiatric problems we see in children, if one traces back the history, one will come to a point at which the diagnosis of an *adjustment reaction* would have been justified. [Jenkins, p. 22]

The second edition of the *Diagnostic and Statistical Manual of Mental Disorders* (DSM-II) endeavored to resolve this classification problem by including a new category–"behavior disorders of childhood and adolescence"–which is taken from the *Eighth Revision of the International Classification of Diseases*. According to the DSM-II (1968): "This major category is reserved for disorders occurring in childhood and adolescence that are more stable, internalized and resistant to treatment than *Transient situational disturbances* . . . but less so than *Psychoses, Neuroses* and *Personality disorders* . . . this intermediate stability is attributed to the greater fluidity of all behavior at this age" (American Psychiatric Association, 1968, p. 50).

The characteristics of six specific types of behavior disorders were summarized under "Behavior Disorders of Childhood and Adolescence" in the DSM-II: hyperkinetic reaction, withdrawing reaction, overanxious reaction, runaway reaction, unsocialized aggressive reaction, and group delinquent reaction. Nailbiting was not mentioned under any of these categories, which perhaps raises the issue "Is fingernail biting in itself considered to be a childhood behavior disorder?" This appears questionable, unless perhaps the nailbiting were very severe and persistent. A seventh category of childhood and adolescent behavior disorders in the DSM-II is an unspecified one called "other reactions of childhood," into which nailbiting could possibly be placed if it were considered a behavior disorder. The DSM-II describes the seventh category as follows: "Here are to be classified children and adolescents having disorders not described in this group but which are nevertheless more serious than transient situational disturbances and less serious than psychoses, neuroses, and personality disorders. The particular disorder should be specified" (American Psychiatric Association, 1968, p. 51).

Recent correspondence with H. H. Work, Deputy Medical Director of the American Psychiatric Association, revealed that nailbiting is not classified in the DSM-III (Work, personal communication). He stated in his letter: "I have searched through the DSM-III and find no particular mention of nailbiting behavior. I assume that it is considered to be merely a symptom of a general anxiety reaction."

Nailbiting was indexed in Volume 2 of the World Health Organization's *Manual of the International Statistical Classification of Diseases, Injuries, and Causes of Death* (World Health Organization, 1978, p. 336) and was included in Section 307 of Volume 1–"Special symptoms or syndromes not elsewhere classified" (p. 201). The symptoms in this classification do not include symptoms "due to mental disorders" or symptoms "of organic origin." Nailbiting was specifically mentioned in Subsection 307.9–"Other and unspecified" items (p. 204). The items listed in this specific category "are not indicative of psychiatric disorder and are included only because such terms may sometimes still appear as diagnoses" (World Health Organization, p. 204). It is somewhat puzzling that nailbiting was included in the chapter of the *Manual of the International Statistical Classification of Diseases, Injuries, and Causes of Death* entitled "Mental Disorders," in view of the characteristics of the category in which it is listed; i.e., that it is not a symptom "due to mental disorders" (p. 201) and "not indicative of psychiatric disorder" (p. 204). In the 1967-69 edition of the *Manual of the International Statistical Classification of Diseases, Injuries, and Causes of Death*, there appeared to be less incongruence in the classification of nailbiting. It was included in the category "behavior disorders of childhood" (World Health Organization, 1967-1969, Vol. 1, p. 152) in the chapter entitled "Mental Disorders."

Nailbiting was also indexed in the American Medical Association's *Standard Nomenclature of Diseases and Operations* (Thompson and Hayden, 1961, p. 734). It was included in the section entitled "Supplementary Terms–Topographic Systems: O to X" and was specifically designated by the code "031" (Thompson and Hayden, 1961, p. 485). In the AMA's *Standard Nomenclature*, a 6-digit code is ordinarily assigned to any disease, symptom, or manifestation–e.g., 248-

123. The "first three digits describe the topographic site; the last three, following the hyphen, describe the etiologic agent" (Thompson and Hayden, 1961, p. x). The first of the three topographic numbers represents a particular system of the body, such as the digestive or musculoskeletal system; the other two numbers specify "a definite organ or part of an organ" (Thompson and Hayden, p. x). The first of the three etiologic numbers represents the etiologic group, such as, trauma, disorder of metabolism, circulatory imbalance; the other two numbers specify the etiologic agent.

Since nailbiting was designated by only a 3-digit code, it was not clear whether a topographic or etiologic consideration was indicated. If topographic, the "0" code would represent the "body as a whole (including the psyche and the body generally) not a particular system exclusively" (Thompson and Hayden, p. x). If the three numbers were an etiologic code, the "0" would indicate a disease "due to prenatal influence" (p. x). The latter hardly seemed applicable, so it was assumed that the "031" was a topographic code. An inquiry to the American Medical Association for confirmation of this assumption and for information regarding the last two numbers was responded to by C. Fanta, Associate Editor, who commented (Fanta, personal communication):

1. The rationale for the zero designation for nail biting is not the specific action itself but the fact that it is a psychologic manifestation. Thus the initial code number is zero, which places it with diseases of the psyche (whole body description).
2. I do not believe the second and third code numbers of the Supplementary Term Section are meant to represent any category at all.

A number of conclusions can be made from the discussion of the significance and classification of nailbiting. The consensus among most writers of major texts in child psychopathology and psychiatry seems to be that fingernail biting is not in itself an important psychiatric symptom unless it is very severe or persistent. Nailbiting is generally acknowledged as an outlet for anxiety. Whether or not nailbiting is problematic depends on the nailbiter's personal reactions and the reaction of friends and relatives to his habit and the appearance of his nails.

Chronic nailbiting is, however, potentially harmful in a number of ways. Quite apart from the nailbiter having to cope with the "deep-seated problem" interpretation of others, fingernail biting is harmful to dentition and oral hygiene. Chronic nailbiting produces small fractures in the incisal edges of the anterior teeth and gingivitis is associated with the trauma of continued nailbiting. More controversial, however, is the fingernail-biting malocclusion hypothesis. Supporters of this hypothesis argue that the orofacial muscular stresses in fingernail biting are disproportionately focused on the small number of teeth involved in tooth-nail contact. This uneven distribution of stress may contribute to the malpositioning of the teeth. The opposing argument is that nailbiting does not produce malocclusion because the muscular forces produced in nailbiting are similar to those involved in chewing food and, therefore, are harmless. Empirical support for the malocclusion-nailbiting notion would be provided if a greater incidence of malocclusion were found among nailbiters and former nailbiters than among nonnailbiters.

Most writers classify nailbiting simply as a habit, whether it be as a nervous habit, oral habit, or secondary habit disturbance. Although nailbiting has been classified as a tic, several writers have opposed this view because the characteristics of nailbiting behavior clearly distinguish it from a tic. Several of these distinguishing features are that nailbiting is voluntarily omitted, can be interrupted, is not repeated in photographically identical form, and involves two parts of the body.

In the standard medical and psychiatric nomenclatures, nailbiting is either not classified, is inconsistently classified within the same volume, or is very vaguely classified. These nomenclatures, therefore, are not very helpful in assisting the clinician or researcher to classify the nailbiting response.

DESCRIPTION OF NAILBITING

For clarity in the data-taking aspect of their treatment procedures for nailbiting, Perkins and Perkins (1976) provided a detailed description of the act of nailbiting. The following instructions were given to their clients in order to help them to accurately monitor separate occurrences of nailbiting behavior:

> Count each separate time your finger(s) goes into your mouth or touches your lip as one instance of nailbiting. For example, if you put your index finger into your mouth and gnaw on the nail, that would be one instance of nailbiting. If you then put your thumb to your mouth touching your lip but put it back down, that would be another instance. Still another time you might bite a nail for about a minute—you would also count that as one instance of nailbiting. In all you should have three tally marks on your card for those three separate occurrences of nailbiting. [Perkins and Perkins, 1976, p. 3]

According to two other researchers (Vargas and Adesso, 1976), nailbiting, for purposes of self-monitoring, included "not only those occasions in which a biting response was actually performed, but all instances whereby a finger was inserted between the lips in such a way that contact between a fingernail and one or more teeth was established" (p. 323).

Bucher (1968) defined the "violation associated with [nail] biting" (p. 391) as "the act of placing a finger in the mouth or on the lips" (p. 389). No specific definition of nailbiting was provided, but one can probably assume in extending beyond this description of the nailbiting violation that fingernail biting would be defined as "the act of placing a finger in the mouth or on the lips" (p. 389) and "actual[ly] biting" (Bucher, personal communication) the free edge of the nail.

In a study by McNamara (1972) of the effect of different self-recording procedures on the nailbiting response, one group of subjects was instructed to record "the nailbiting response if it occurred," but no definition of this response was provided in the study. Each subject in another group was asked "to engage in a resistance response by pulling [his] hand away from [his] mouth every time [his] fingers touched [his] lips and to self-record this behavior" (p. 193). A definition of nailbiting appears to be inherent in this description of the resistance response: "Every time [his] fingers touched [his] lips." It is interesting to note that a similar response was the target behavior in the investigation by Bucher (1968). Billig reported that he had unobtrusively observed the nailbiting activity of 10th-grade girls. During his observations he was able to note and subsequently outline four basic components of the response chain of nailbiting:

> (a) The placing of one hand in the vicinity of the mouth. This posture continues from a few seconds to half a minute. (b) The placing of a finger against the teeth. This step is usually accomplished very rapidly. (c) A series of quick, spasmodic bitings, with the nail of the finger pressed tightly against the biting edge of the teeth. (d) This step consists of the withdrawal of the finger from the mouth, to be inspected either visually or to be felt by another finger or by the other hand. The facial expression at this period is rather serious. If the biter becomes aware of being watched the proceeding is abruptly brought to an end. The entire sequence lasts anywhere from about 40 seconds to several minutes. [Billig, 1941, pp. 162-163]

Fingernail biting as defined by Nunn and Azrin (1976) included "any hand movements which resulted in damage to the nails or cuticles and skin area surrounding the nails" (p. 65). This definition is puzzling because it could refer to the behavior of nail-picking as well as to nailbiting. In their book entitled *Habit Control in a Day*, Azrin and Nunn (1977) defined nail-picking as "using the thumb to pick at the other fingers of the same hand" or as picking "at the fingers and thumb of one hand with the thumb of the other hand" (p. 53). These two patterns of nail-picking both involve hand movements and hence could be included in Nunn and Azrin's (1976) definition of nailbiting. Another statement by Azrin and Nunn (1977) that seemed to favor the inclusion of nail-picking in their definition of nailbiting was that "the person usually picks at the nail for a period of time, then begins biting" (p. 53). The nail-picking aspect of this sequence appears to be a habit-associated activity, which Azrin and Nunn (1977) defined as movements that "precede the habit movement in such a way that a regular sequence can be seen" (p. 48). Nail-picking, therefore, may be regarded as a nailbiting-associated movement. Habit-associated movements were regarded as "integral parts of the habit" (Azrin and Nunn, 1977, p. 51), which may lead one to conclude that nail-picking is an integral part of nailbiting. If this is so, and since both nailbiting and nail-picking involve hand movements, it is difficult to determine whether or not the definition of nailbiting in the article by Nunn and Azrin (1976) included nail-picking.

Samman (1972) commented on the nature of nailbiting behavior:

> All finger-nails are often bitten, but occasionally one or more is spared. The nail is often bitten right back to its point of separation from its bed. Fine spicules may be left at the edge which cause splits and mild paronychia. Concurrently with the biting of the nail the cuticles are often bitten, and so become irregular and broken. . . . Hang nails . . .due to small hard pieces of epidermis breaking away from the lateral nail folds . . . [are] often due to nail biting. [pp. 1659-1660]

A definite order of finger preference in biting among children aged 5-18 years was revealed in a study by Malone and Massler (1952). As reported in their investigation, "The nailbiter usually began with the thumb, advanced to the index finger, skipped to the little finger, thence to the middle finger, and last to the ring finger" (p. 201). Malone and Massler did not account for this systematic preference, but they provided a rationale for the ring finger being ranked last in terms of preference for biting. They explained that separation of the ring finger from the others is hindered by the nature of its ligamentous attachments, which makes the biting of this finger rather awkward for the child (p. 201). Malone and Massler reported that 96.7% of the nailbiters in their study showed no preference for left or right hand as determined by analysis of data for hand and finger preference in biting. This finding of bilateral symmetry was interpreted by Malone and Massler to probably indicate "that nailbiting is an *unconscious* activity" (p. 201).

Anatomy and Growth Rate of the Fingernail

ANATOMICAL DESCRIPTION OF THE FINGERNAIL

As illustrated in Figures 2 and 3, the nail consists of the nail plate and the tissues which surround and underlie it (Pillsbury, Shelley, and Kligman, 1956, p. 32). The nail plate is composed of hard keratin, a protein that is synthesized by the nail-forming tissue called the *matrix*. The average daily rate of linear nail growth is approximately .1 mm (Morton, 1962; Norton, 1975; Pillsbury et al., 1956); this nail-forming tissue is in a highly active metabolic state and is very sensitive to local or generalized physiological alterations, such as trauma to the nails, localized infection, or disease. The nail plate itself is an inert structure that consists of three main parts: (a) the root, which is beneath the skin; (b) the fixed portion, which is firmly attached to the underlying nail bed; (c) the free edge of the nail, which extends beyond the distal-most point of attachment of the nail plate to the nail bed (Pillsbury et al., 1956).

On the proximal area of the nail plate, a semilunar structure called the *lunula* is visible in varying degrees with different individuals and races and also with different fingers within an individual. It is usually present and most noticeable on the thumbnail, whereas it may be totally absent on the little finger. The lunula actually represents the anterior portion of the matrix of the nail, which can be determined

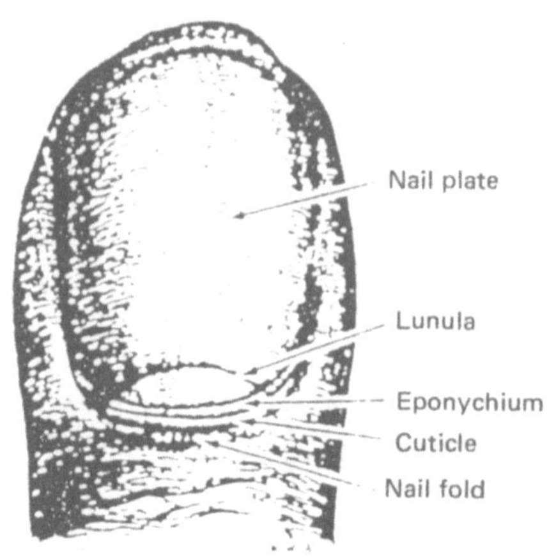

Figure 2 Nail. From *Synopsis of dermatology* (2d ed.), by W. D. Stewart, J. L. Danto, and S. Maddin. St. Louis: Mosby, 1970, p. 13. Copyright by C. V. Mosby Co. Ltd.; reprinted with permission.

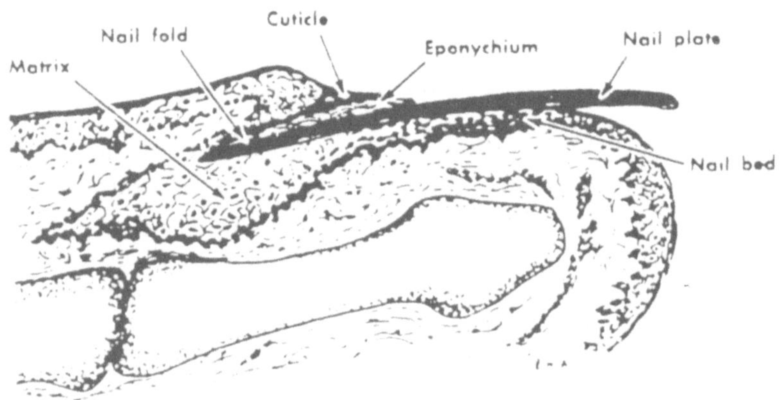

Figure 3 Nail bed, saggital section. From *Synopsis of dermatology* (2d ed.), by W. D. Stewart, J. L. Danto, and S. Maddin. St. Louis: Mosby, 1970, p. 13. Copyright by C. V. Mosby Co. Ltd.; reprinted with permission.

by a comparison of Figures 2 and 3. The boundary between the lunula's two underlying structures, the matrix and the nail bed, is represented by the distal convex line formed by the lunula (Pillsbury et al., 1956).

The keratinization that occurs continuously in the matrix is responsible for the white color of the lunula. The rest of the nail plate is pinkish because of the rich arterial blood supply in the underlying nail bed (Pillsbury et al.). It was once believed that nail formation was solely the function of the matrix but, according to Stewart, Danto, and Maddin (1970, p. 13), the nail bed does appear to participate.

A yellowish-pink or brownish-pink band may be observed near the free edge of the nail. This band marks the point where the nail bed begins to become continuous with the epidermis of the finger. This means that essentially the nail bed is being converted at this point to a keratin-producing membrane. The whitish substance that often accumulates under the free edge is loose keratin, a resultant product of the transformation that occurs at the point of separation of the nail plate from the nail bed. Due to this process, the nail bed becomes continuous with the epidermis of the finger but the nail plate continues to extend in length indefinitely unless cut or worn away through use (Pillsbury et al.).

The nail plate is inserted into grooves, which are bounded by nail folds, both laterally and posteriorly. The nail folds contain cells that produce soft keratin, which adheres to the nail plate as a tough membrane called the *eponychium* (see Figures 2 and 3). This membrane extends forward as the nail grows. The posterior nail fold contributes the greatest amount of eponychium, but some is also deposited by the lateral nail folds and can be evident on the nail plate (Pillsbury et al., 1956).

The *cuticle* is a "flattened, elastic, keratinous rim" (Pillsbury et al., p. 35) at the anterior border of the posterior nail fold which functions as a protective structure for the nail fold. Usually the eponychium and the cuticle are manipulated during manicuring.

SOURCES OF VARIATION IN FINGERNAIL GROWTH RATES

Fingernail growth begins during the early stages of fetal development. A classic article entitled "Drama of Life Before Birth" in the April 30th, 1965 issue of *Life* photographically depicts the presence of fingernails in a 16-week-old fetus. The nails are often long enough to enable the fetus to actually "put quite a number of scratches on its face before it is born" (p. 68).

Babcock (1955) noted that although body growth in general is a slow process, the nails "grow at relatively rapid rates in all animals, large and small, young and old" (p. 324). In a recent dermatology text, Norton (1975) stated that the fingernails grow at a rate of approximately .1 mm a day with little variation. Bean (1953, 1963) reported the results of a 20-year (N = 1) study of the growth of his own left thumbnail. The data revealed: no seasonal variation in the rate of growth; no effect on growth by factors such as geographical location, occupation, or physical activity; and "slow or interrupted growth" (Bean, 1953, p. 29) of the nail during an acute illness. Bean (1953) confined his measurements to the left thumbnail because in an earlier series of studies, he had found "no great variability in rate of growth of any of the individual nails of the hand" (p. 27).

The comprehensive study of nail growth in a large population by Hamilton, Terada, and Mestler (cited in Bean, 1963) showed that "increased metabolism is associated with [an] increased rate of nail growth. This is shown in pregnancy where the rate of growth may be increased by as much as one-third" (p. 480), and during the time when rapid acceleration in adolescent growth occurs. The Hamilton et al. study also showed that the rate of nail growth is slightly greater in males than in females.

Basler (cited in Babcock, 1955) reported that nighttime nail growth was slower than daytime growth. He suggested that this may be due to the reduced blood pressure when an individual is asleep, and hence the reduced blood flow to the nail bed. Similarly, Weir and Mitchell's study in 1871 revealed that fingernail growth was retarded in paralyzed hands (Babcock, 1955, p. 327) and was resumed just prior to the return of motor activity. Babcock (1955) also made reference to the work of Head and Sherren, who in 1908 had observed a similar retardation of nail growth when the hand was immobilized in a splint or cast, but noted that massage stimulated the growth (Babcock, p. 327). Interesting from a historical point of view and consistent with these observations is the finding by Blake in 1899 that "the rate of nail growth is normal in hysterical paralysis" (cited in Bean, 1963, p. 479).

With regard to the reported retardation in nail growth during certain diseases and illnesses, Morton (1962) pointed out that "although it can be established in certain cases that there is a retardation of growth below the average normal rate, a conclusive result presupposes a knowledge of the patient's normal rate of nail growth before the onset of the disease" (p. 28).

Several studies have given indications that fluctuations occur in the rate of growth of the human fingernail. For example, in a study of nail growth in a group of British naval personnel, Geohegan, Roberts, and Sanford (cited in Bean, 1963) found that while the subjects were stationed in the Arctic, the mean daily growth was .114 mm per day, whereas in the temperate coastal waters of Britain, their nail growth was .1194 mm per day (p. 481). Bean offered an explanation for the seasonal variation in nail growth and also provided his rationale for the absence of any seasonal variation in the growth of his own thumbnail:

> By far the simplest explanation for this observation is that in temperate climates there is a greater degree of cutaneous vasodilatation; in cold environments the temperature regulating machinery of the skin reduces blood flow and thus the growth of cutaneous appendages is reduced. My own failure to produce changes in growth with the seasons probably reflects the fact that the average exposure to very cold weather rarely amounted to more than a half hour a day, and the rest of the time was spent inside centrally heated buildings. [Bean, 1963, p. 481]

Taking measurements from the lunula of the nail with an illuminated magnifying glass, Clark and Buxton (cited in Babcock, 1955) found that "growth was essentially the same for left and right thumbs, for male and female, and for ages 10 to 23 years, but . . . it was greater in the summer and for nail-biters, and . . . there was wide variation between individuals" (p. 325). Pillsbury et al. (1956) concurred with these reports, stating that nail growth is accelerated with "elevation of the environmental temperature and as a result of occupational trauma or nail biting" (p. 38).

Although Bean (1963) found no seasonal variation in the growth rate of his thumbnail, he noted slight changes with increasing age. At the age of 32, the average daily rate of growth was .123 mm. At age 42, it was .111 mm, and at age 52, .105 mm. Bean (1963) noted that at age 49, a sharp decline in growth rate was evident, which at the time of his 52nd year seemed to be continuing. Hamilton et al. (cited in Lavelle, 1968) also reported a decrease in the rate of nail growth with advancing age. They concluded, however, that since the thickness of the nails increased, "the actual volume of growth remained virtually stable" (Lavelle, p. 557).

Gilchrist and Buxton (cited in Babcock, 1955) studied the relation of fingernail growth to nutrition in different groups of young schoolchildren. They found "a highly significant difference in fingernail growth rates between children rated as having 'subnormal' nutrition, and those rated as 'normal' or as 'excellent' but no significant difference between the 'normal' and 'excellent' groups (Babcock, 1955, p. 325). Their clinical ratings of nutritional status were based on general physical appearance rather than on specific symptoms associated with nutritional deficits (Babcock, 1955). The clinical ratings, therefore, "may have been influenced by factors that had little effect on fingernail growth" (Babcock, p. 326) and this may have accounted for the small differences in the rates of nail growth among the three groups of children in the Gilchrist and Buxton investigation.

One researcher systematically assessed the effect of cosmetic nail-covering on nail growth. In an N = 1 study by Morton (1962), "the great toe-nail of the left foot was coated, while that of the right acted as a control." Morton found that "although the varnish caused disruption of the nail surface, it did not affect growth in comparison with the uncoated nail; the growth rate remained constant over the nail surface" (p. 28).

MEASUREMENT OF THE RATE OF NAIL GROWTH

Babcock (1955) has stressed that in short-term studies, quantitative assessments of nail growth cannot be conveniently made because of the small changes in linear growth that occur on a daily basis. Nails "grow at the rate of about 0.1 mm per day; this distance is so small" that magnification may be necessary to obtain accurate readings (p. 327).

Babcock cautioned that obtaining quantitative measurements of nail growth in long-term studies also may present several problems, noting that there is evidence in the literature to indicate that "fingernail formation is probably influenced by the state of nutrition, endocrine factors, disease, and environmental factors" (p. 335). In view of the difficulty of controlling extraneous variables as the duration of the experimental period increases, Babcock concluded that "methods for measuring nail growth over short time periods are to be preferred" (p. 334), despite the inconvenience of having to use magnification procedures.

One of the more suitable methods of measuring linear nail growth, as suggested by Babcock, is the photographic method. According to Babcock (p. 327), taking photographs of the subject's fingernails appears to have three advantages over other methods that employ direct measurements on live subjects. Photographs (a) furnish a permanent record of the length of the nail at a particular point in time, (b) allow for rapid data collection (some procedures may be cumbersome and time-consuming), and (c) permit optical enlargement of the distance to be measured.

Bean (1953) asserted that fingernail growth may be measured in a number of ways. One of these techniques involves indelibly staining the nail with a substance such as nitric acid. Another involves making a scratch on the nail with a sharp instrument, which was the method used by Bean in measuring the linear nail growth of his left thumb over a period of 20 years. Specifically, he reported that he scored the nail "sharply . . . exactly where it emerged from beneath the cuticle" (p. 27).

A third method suggested by Bean (1953) is to measure or weigh "clippings from the nail" (p. 27). One cautionary note from Bean concerning this method is that it is usually rendered inaccurate by the natural wearing away of the terminal portion of the nail.

It seems that using measurements taken from fingernail clippings would be unsatisfactory as a dependent variable to assess the efficacy of nailbiting treatments on either a short-term or long-term basis. In short-term studies, for example, the nail plate of severely bitten nails would not have sufficient time to attain a free edge from which clippings could be taken. Especially significant in long-term studies is the obvious problem to be encountered with taking regular measurements from severely bitten fingernails. Graphically, progress in treatment and nail growth would be depicted in a distorted manner since no nail growth could be graphed until the nail plate had a free edge. The point at which a graph illustrates growth of the nail would not reflect the actual beginning of growth, but only its beginning as determined by this procedure. In the case of very severe nailbiters, therefore, this technique would considerably underestimate the total amount of linear growth of the nail plate. Practically speaking, if reinforcement were made strictly contingent on nail growth as assessed by this method, the severe nailbiter would be deprived of reinforcement in the early stages of treatment.

Babcock, noted that measuring an increase in the length of nails involves measuring the distance between a mark on the nail and a reference point on the finger (1955, p. 327). He enumerated a number of problems that are likely to be encountered in obtaining a suitable reference point:

> The greatest problem in measuring fingernail growth is the choice of a reference point for the measurements. The cuticle, used by early workers, is inaccurate for short-term studies because it can easily be pressed back. The same applies to the point of separation of the nail from its bed. The lunula frequently is not visible on all fingers and does not appear as a sharp line when viewed through the nail with a magnifying glass. It does not show clearly on ordinary photographs, and it is said to be affected by pathologic changes that affect the nails or nail bed. . . . In the studies reported here, three reference points have been tested, the phalanx bone, the skin near the nail, and the lunula. [pp. 327-328]

The area of the finger from which Babcock determined a reference point for his assessment of linear growth by ordinary photographic means was the "skin between the nail and the terminal finger joint." He added that "the reference point could be either a mark made on the skin, or the small skin wrinkles in this area." After the photographs were taken, they were read by "superimposing the images of the skin wrinkles and measuring the distance the mark on the nail had advanced" (Babcock, p. 328).

The reference point that was used for taking measurements by means of x-ray photographs was the terminal finger bone. A deep scratch was made on the nail and it was filled with bismuth amalgam, a material that is opaque to x-rays (Babcock, 1955). An x-ray photograph was taken of the finger before and after a 41-day growth period. The images of the terminal finger bone in the two photographs were exactly superimposed, which enabled the distance between the "before" and "after" positions of the scratch mark to be measured. This technique is depicted in Figure 4.

Babcock compared the accuracy of measurements taken from x-ray photographs and those taken from ordinary photographs. The

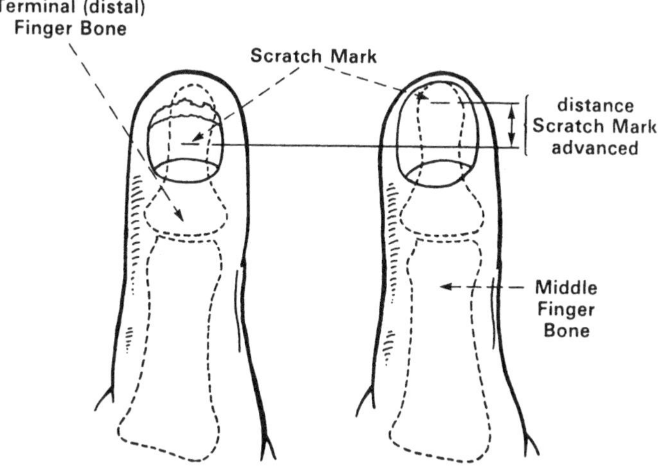

Figure 4 Babcock's x-ray method of measuring fingernail growth.

results of this comparison of the two photographic methods revealed that there was "virtually no bias or inaccuracy in the [ordinary] photographic method, using the x-ray method as an absolute reference for measuring growth" over a period of at least a month (pp. 329-330).

Babcock further investigated the skin photographic method of linear nail growth measurement by attempting to determine its effectiveness when adapted to short-term studies of one week's duration. In order to facilitate measurement over such a short period of time, "the small distance that the scratch-mark image advanced was increased . . . by taking enlarged photographs (6.4X) of a single finger" (Babcock, p. 330). Two photographs were taken at the beginning of the study and two at the end of the growth period in order to provide "a measure of variation caused by positioning the finger" (p. 330). The details provided by Babcock (1955) for setting up the camera and taking the photographs follow:

> The camera was prefocused on a three-fourths inch square opening in a firmly mounted piece of sheet metal, and the finger was gently pressed upward against this frame. The illumination was standardized by clamping two 375-watt reflector-type photoflood bulbs 8 inches from the frame. The exposure (two seconds at f:22) was controlled by an automatic timer switch connected

> to the lights. Two photographs were taken at the beginning of the growth period, and two photographs were made at the end of one week. Replicate growth measurements were thus obtained, one from each pair of photographs. [p. 330]

Results of this investigation led Babcock to report that "the skin-photographic method did not have the desired degree of precision when used with short growth periods" (p. 331).

Using the ordinary photographic method, Babcock attempted to ascertain if another part of the nail, the lunula, would be a suitable reference point for measuring nail growth. The thumbnail was selected for study because the lunula of this nail "is usually more distinct than that of the other fingernails" (Babcock, p. 331). Adjustment of photographic conditions allowed for maximum contrast of the lunula.

In preparation of the thumbnail for photographing, a light scratch was made near the lunula and was filled with a red pigment. The nail was then pressed upward against a firmly mounted microscopic slide. Glycerol was first applied to the nail so as to minimize reflections from its surface. Care was also taken to retain maximum contrast of the lunula with the nail while pressing against the slide; too much pressure would push the blood out of the nail bed and hence reduce the contrast of the lunula with the rest of the nail. Photographs were taken under identical conditions before and after a 1-week time interval. Using the negatives, the before and after images of the lunula were superimposed and the distance between the two scratch marks was measured "with a microscope ocular micrometer scale containing 140 divisions in 8.4 mm and a 7.5X magnifying glass" (Babcock, p. 332). After separating the negatives, Babcock read them four more times and "the average of the 5 readings was converted to microns of growth per day" (Babcock, p. 332). Tests revealed that it was easier to align a negative with a positive transparency than with another negative. In Babcock's study, the increased precision and ease in reading the transparencies made it possible to detect approximately a 5% difference in linear nail growth.

The photographic method that used skin wrinkles as a reference point did not provide as accurate a measurement as either of the two lunula methods, since the skin was distorted when the finger contacted the focusing frame of the camera. Babcock explained the advantages of using the lunula as a reference point:

> [The lunula] appears to be a relatively stable reference point for short-term studies. Slight variations in the edge of the lunula would have little effect on the readings because the negatives are placed in register by superimposing the two images of the entire lunula, rather than by measuring from a specific point on the edge of the lunula. The greater precision of the lunula methods makes them preferable to the skin-photographic method for short-term studies. With subjects whose lunula is indistinct, however, the skin-photographic method could be applied, preferably with a growth period longer than one week to increase precision. [pp. 333-334]

Morton (1962) used a modified form of Babcock's superimposition method of measuring linear nail growth. Whereas most other techniques provided an assessment of the rate of growth of the entire nail, Morton's method allowed for further refinement in measurement. He was able to determine "whether the normal nail grows at the same rate peripherally as centrally and whether the nail growth is constant from base to tip" (Morton, p. 27). Several writers have used the lunula as a reference point, but according to Morton this method is open to suspicion since the lunula "is often ill defined and in many cases absent" (p. 26).

Morton's technique involved drilling several small holes in the nail plate with a "No. 80 (0.0135 in.) twist drill in a thumb-chuck" (p. 27). These holes did not penetrate the nail plate, but were deep enough to be filled with black crayon wax. This provided a permanent method of marking the nail. After the photographs were taken, the negatives were enlarged and the position of the main skin wrinkles and drilled holes were marked on an underlying card. The images of the skin creases in succeeding negatives could be placed exactly over the lines on the card that represented these creases and then the distance between the drilled holes could be measured.

In his study of the consistency of the rate of growth of the nail, Morton (1962) drilled two parallel rows of five holes across the nail plate (see Figure 5). The rationale for drilling two rows of holes rather than a single hole was that this technique would allow for measurement of growth at several points on the nail. After a 12-week period, during which the thumbnail was photographed once a week, Morton found that the first and last negatives could be superimposed exactly (the rows of drilled holes could be exactly aligned), as illustrated in Figure 5, indicating that "growth along and at right angles to the long axis of the nail was constant" (p. 28). An inspection of the plotted data (see Figure 6) reveals that linear nail growth appeared to regularly increase at a rate of approximately .1 mm per day during the course of the 12-week period of the study.

Kandil (1972) described a method that is suitable for either short-term or long-term studies under conditions in which "nail growth is slower than normal" (p. 55). In Kandil's x-ray marker technique, a thin, narrow brass tape (approximately 1.12 mm wide and .06 mm thick) in the shape of an arrow is glued with a chemically reactive adhesive to the surface of the nail plate. Basically, the procedure involves taking an antero-posterior x-ray from the palm side of the hand of the distal two phalanges, so that the brass arrow appears clearly on the film. After several weeks, another x-ray is taken under identical conditions, namely, "36-inch distance, 100 ma; 0.10' time and 50 kv" (Kandil, p. 54).

If a measurement of nail growth over a short time period is required, the second x-ray may be taken after only 1 week and adjustments made in the measuring technique so that an estimate of 4

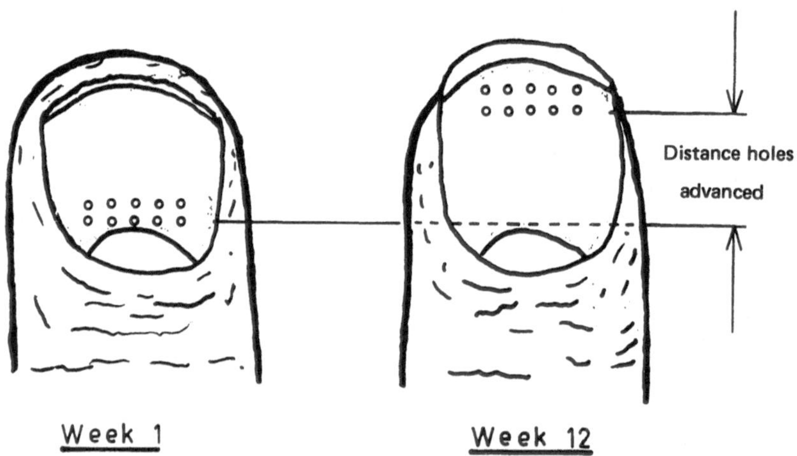

Figure 5 Photographic hole-drilling technique of measuring fingernail growth. Adapted from "Visual Assessment of Nail Growth," by R. Morton, *Medical and Biological Illustration*, 1962, *12*, 26-30. Copyright by Medical and Biological Illustration; reprinted with permission.

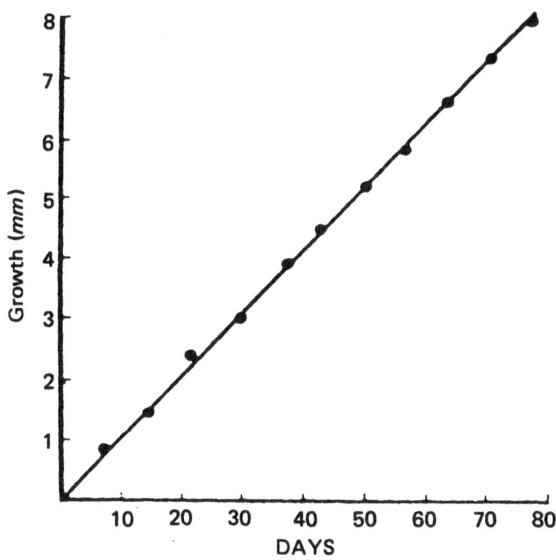

Figure 6 Growth rate curve of a normal adult thumb nail. From "Visual Assessment of Nail Growth," by R. Morton, *Medical and Biological Illustration*, 1962, *12*, 26-30. Copyright by Medical and Biological Illustration; reprinted with permission.

weeks' growth can be made. Kandil recommended the following procedure:

> The x-ray films are enlarged four times onto positive paper; this procedure is by no means a difficult one for any trained photographer. The measurement obtained after this enlargement corresponds to four weeks' growth . . . and should be taken with a compass since errors in measurement are exaggerated four times. [p. 54]

Antero-posterior x-rays rather than postero-anterior exposures (taken from the back side of the hand) were used by Kandil because he felt that a postero-anterior exposure "carries the most unavoidable risk of axial rotation of the fingers during x-ray photography" (p. 56). He recognized, however, that if postero-anterior exposures could be used, they would have the advantage of minimizing any possibility of magnification.

MEASUREMENT TECHNIQUES USED IN BEHAVIORAL STUDIES OF NAILBITING

Stephen and Konig recognized that nailbiting is "a useful response paradigm in behavior therapy studies because it . . . [can be] reliably observed and measured" (1970, p. 211). Simple observation of the symptom or damage to the fingernails is generally used as a guideline for identifying those individuals who would qualify as potential subjects for studying the behavioral aspects of nailbiting. Specific criteria that have been suggested by R. G. Nunn for diagnosing fingernail biting and its associated movements are that "nail-biting and nail-picking are identified by the partial or complete absence of nails, or by roughened skin area surrounding the nail" (1978, p. 350).

Some exploratory studies, such as Bucher's investigation, contained no measures of fingernail length because of the ease with which fingernail biting could be observed. In this study, subjects were individually instructed to record the frequency of self-administered shocks contingent on "placing a finger in the mouth or on the lips" (1968, p. 389). Neither a rating scale nor a physical measure of nail length was used but visual checks of the subjects' nails were made by the experimenter and used to corroborate the subjects' self-report measures.

Many researchers have incorporated measurement techniques into their studies. For example, Stephen and Koenig photographed the hands of their subjects and measured each subject's fingernails prior to their study and took measurements twice-weekly thereafter for five weeks. A micrometer was used to determine nail length, as measured from "the base of the nail to the longest portion of the nail" (1970, p. 211). Each measurement of fingernail length, taken at regular intervals during the investigation and expressed in hundredths of an inch, was compared with the measurement taken on the previous inspection. There was no indication that reliability checks were employed.

During the course of a 4-week study by McNamara (1972), fingernail length was measured in fiftieths of an inch by using a special ruler: "Nail length was measured from the base of the nail, at a point which separated skin from cuticle, to the center-most portion of the top of the nail" (p. 193). Inter-rater reliability of the measurements was determined.

Vargas and Adesso (1976) measured nail length "from the base of the nail at the point where it separated from the cuticle to the center-most portion of the top of the nail. The individual lengths of the 10 fingernails were then summed to yield a composite nail-length measure for each subject" (p. 323). Vargas and Adesso stressed, however, that measurement of increases in nail length may be inappropriate as a dependent variable to evaluate certain treatment techniques. With reference to negative practice,* they stated:

> A problem inherent to negative practice is that it can have a direct effect on nail length. Should an individual actually bite his nails rather than gnaw on them while engaged in negative practice, evaluation of the technique would be biased. [Vargas and Adesso, p. 327]

Horan, Hoffman, and Macri (1974) based their nailbiting assessment procedure not only on nail length but on the cosmetic appearance of the nails. Fingernail length was assessed "to the nearest 1/64th in. from the top center of the nail to a point which separated the bottom center of the cuticle and the skin" (p. 307). They subjectively determined a "cosmetic appearance score . . . by counting the number of fingers showing cuticle disfigurement and adding to this quantity, the number of fingers with traces of blood or scabs" (Horan et al., p. 308).

Malone and Massler's (1952) analytic formulation provides the only systematic procedure to appear in the psychological literature to date for defining and assessing the degree of fingernail biting. Unlike most studies, their "Index of Nailbiting in Children" differentiated between mild, moderate, and severe nailbiting and provided a means of evaluating the nailbiter according to the number of fingernails bitten and the degree or severity of the biting.

With regard to the number of fingernails bitten, Malone and Massler categorized the children in their study as *nonnailbiters, definite nailbiters,* or *indefinite nailbiters* (p. 194). They defined nonnailbiters as those children who do not bite any of their fingernails; definite nailbiters were those children who bite all 10 fingernails, and indefinite

*Upon instructions from the experimenter, subjects were asked to engage in nailbiting behavior (without actually biting) for 10 uninterrupted minutes at each session, one minute per finger. Six experimental sessions were arranged for each subject on approximately a weekly basis. Subjects were also asked to engage in the nailbiting behavior for three minutes each evening.

nailbiters were children who bite 1 to 9 fingernails. They referred to the indefinite nailbiters as perhaps being "transitional between the other two categories" (p. 194).

According to Malone and Massler's (1952) scale of measurement, each finger may be given a rating of 0, 1+, 2+, or 3+. Zero indicates that the fingernails are not bitten; 1+, that they are mildly bitten; 2+, that they are moderately bitten; 3+, that they are severely bitten. The quantitative and descriptive aspects of the scale are summarized in Table 2 and illustrated in Figure 7. The ratings for the 10 fingernails were summed to provide an index. Hence, a child may have an index of nailbiting ranging from 0 to 30. For example, a "definite nailbiter" (one who bites all 10 fingernails) who has a severity rating of 2+ for all 10 fingers would have an index of 20 (10 × 2+). A child who bit five fingernails at the 1+ degree of severity would have an index of 5 (5 × 1+). According to Malone and Massler, there is considerable evidence for a positive correlation between the number of fingernails bitten and the severity of the nailbiting. They based their claim on two observations from their investigation. Irrespective of the sex of the nailbiter, they found that:

1. Indefinite biters (1 to 9 fingernails bitten) showed mild degrees of nailbiting severity. They bit "to an index from 1 to 10" (Malone and Massler, p. 198) on the nailbiting scale of severity.

Table 2 A Scale for Measuring the Severity of Fingernail Biting

Degree of fingernail biting	*Description*
0 (not bitten)	Free margin intact.
1+ (mildly bitten)	Free edge of nail irregular but reasonably intact. Fingernail biting confirmed on questioning.[a]
2+ (moderately bitten)	Free margin of nail absent. Regular biting confirmed on questioning.
3+ (severely bitten)	Fingernail bitten beyond the free edge; nail margin below the soft tissue border (Fig. 7).

From "Index of Nailbiting in Children" by A. J. Malone and M. Massler, *Journal of Abnormal and Social Psychology*, 1952, *47*, 193-202. Copyright by the American Psychological Association and reprinted with permission.

[a]In cases of doubt, the fingernail was assumed to have been accidentally broken and was not scored as bitten. This seldom occurred.

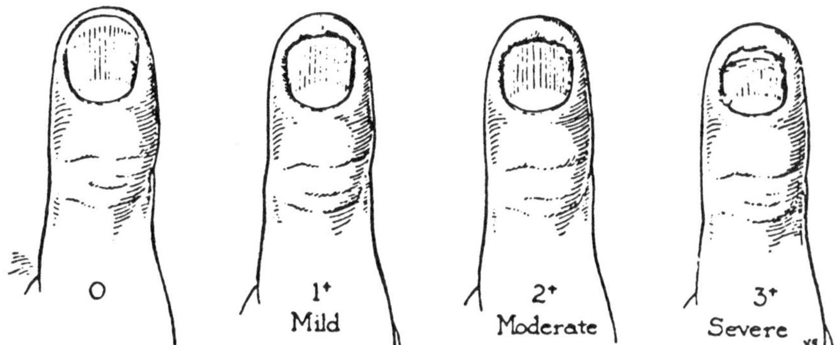

Figure 7 Diagram showing different degrees of fingernail biting. From "Index of Nailbiting in Children," by A. J. Malone and M. Massler, *Journal of Abnormal and Social Psychology*, 1952, *47*, 193-202. Copyright by the American Psychological Association; reprinted with permission.

2. Definite nailbiters (children who bite 10 fingernails) tended with few exceptions to bite at an index from 11 to 30. In fact, 57% of the definite nailbiters bit at an index of 30.

Smith (1957) employed a modified version of the Malone and Massler scale for rating the degree of fingernail biting. In view of Malone and Massler's finding that most of their subjects who bit their fingernails bit all ten with the same degree of severity, each of the fingernails of the subjects in Smith's study was "inspected carefully and then a composite rating of 0, 1, 2, or 3 recorded" (p. 221). These overall scores were based on the Malone and Massler classification in that a score of 0 meant "not bitten"; 1 meant "mildly bitten"; 2 signified "moderately bitten"; and 3 meant "severely bitten." Smith recognized, however, that his procedure was not sensitive to the differences in biting severity among a subject's fingernails. For example, a subject who had three nonbitten and seven severely bitten fingernails would receive a score of 3, because most of his fingernails were severely bitten; an individual who had bitten all 10 fingernails severely would also receive a score of 3. Malone and Massler's more sensitive scale, however, would reflect the obvious difference in the degree of fingernail biting between the two individuals. According to their method of assessment, the scores would be 21 for the subject who bit 7 fingernails severely (7 × 3) and 30 for the subject who bit 10 fingernails severely (10 × 3).

3

Age, Sex, Personality, Intelligence, and Sociological Variables

AGE AND SEX TRENDS

Nailbiting was one of the developmental problems discussed in a monograph by Macfarlane, Allen, and Honzik (1954). This report was based on the data obtained in the longitudinal Berkeley Guidance Study, a landmark in the investigation of developmental problems of normal children from the age of 21 months to 14 years. Clarizio and McCoy (1976) summarized several developmental patterns that were revealed by the Macfarlane et al. (1954) study:

> The problems, which declined with age, were (1) elimination controls (enuresis and soiling), (2) fears, (3) thumb-sucking, (4) destructiveness, and (5) temper outbursts. Only one problem, nailbiting, increased with age, although this too was beginning to drop off by age 14. [pp. 5; 7]

Malone and Massler (1952) found that 41% of the 4,587 children in their survey were nailbiters; they were considered as such on the basis of their having bitten one or more of their fingernails. Twenty-eight percent of the children in the survey bit all 10 fingernails (68% of the nailbiters) and hence were classified as *definite nailbiters*. Thirteen percent of the total number of children were *indefinite nailbiters*; i.e., they bit from 1 to 9 fingernails. Children who bit mildly constituted 11% of the group; those who bit moderately, 12%; those who bit severely, 18% (see Table 3).

Malone and Massler (1952) commented that the prevalence of nailbiting among 5- to 18-year-old boys and girls as determined in their survey was "higher than that reported by Wechsler in 1931" (p. 200). Wechsler (1931) did not record nailbiting severity, but his observational techniques were essentially the same as those employed by Malone and Massler. Only 28% of the 5- to 6-year-old children in Wechsler's study were nailbiters, whereas Malone and Massler found that 38% of children in this age group bit their fingernails. For the children in Malone and Massler's study, the peak period of nailbiting was "the prepubertal period (8-10 years of age) while Wechsler's group . . . reached its peak at puberty (12-14 years of age)" (Malone and Massler, p. 200). In attempting to account for (a) the greater prevalence of nailbiting among the children in their study at every

Table 3 Distribution of Different Types of Nailbiters. Percentage of Total Number Children

	Nailbiting	
	Number of fingernails bitten	*Degree (index) of fingernail biting*
Non-nailbiters 59%	None	(0)
Nailbiters 41%	Indefinite (1-9 fingers) 13.0%	Mild (1-10) 11%
	Definite (10 fingers) 28.0%	Moderate (11-20) 12.2%
		Severe (21-30) 17.9%

From "Index of Nailbiting in Children," by A. J. Malone and M. Massler, *Journal of Abnormal and Social Psychology*, 1952, *47*, 193-202. Copyright by the American Psychological Association and reprinted with permission.

age level, (b) the greater number of 5- and 6-year-old nailbiters and hence earlier onset of nailbiting, and for (c) the earlier peak periods of nailbiting, Malone and Massler commented: "These differences appear to be real and not accidental and might indicate that tensions in children have increased during the last two decades (1931 to 1950)" (p. 200). A comparison between Wechsler's findings and those of Malone and Massler with regard to nailbiting prevalence is presented in Figure 8.

With regard to age and sex trends, the results of the Malone and Massler survey indicated that "the number of definite (10) nailbiters increased from a low of 28 percent at 5 years of age to a peak of 50

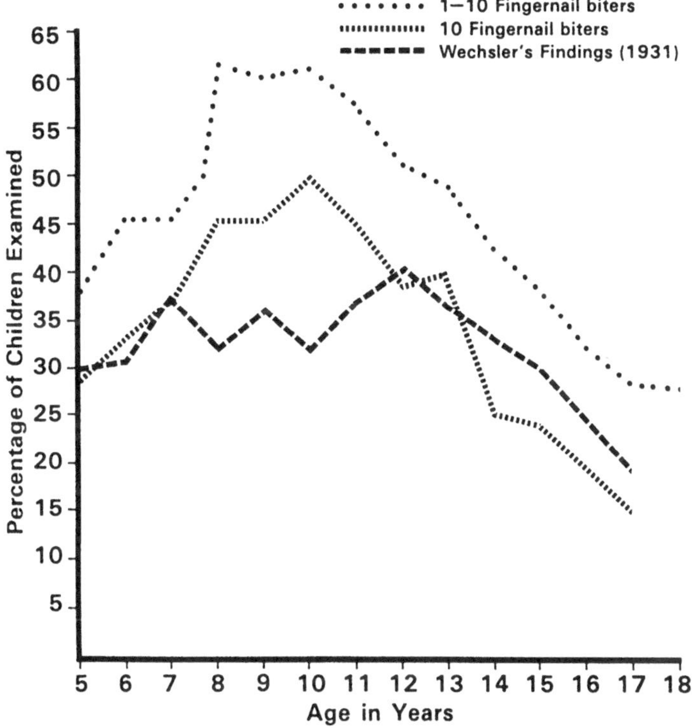

Figure 8 Comparison of prevalence of nailbiting as determined by Wechsler in 1931 with Malone and Massler's 1952 study. Adapted from "Index of Nailbiting in Children," by A. J. Malone, and M. Massler, *Journal of Abnormal and Social Psychology*, 1952, *47*, 193-202. Copyright by the American Psychological Association; reprinted with permission.

per cent at the age of 10 years, decelerating rapidly thereafter to 15 per cent at 18 years of age" (p. 194). No particular age trend was evident among the indefinite nailbiters, which reaffirms, according to Malone and Massler, . . . "the hypothesis that this is an "indefinite" group and one which is probably not significant to the total picture of fingernail biting" (p. 195).

To determine if severity of nailbiting was characterized by age trends, Malone and Massler (1952) graphed the data of children in each of the three categories of severity: mild, moderate, and severe. The graph indicated:

> There is no significant increase or decrease from five to 18 years of age in the number of children who bite their fingernails mildly (index 1-10) or moderately (index 11-20). However, the number of children who bite severely (index 21-30) rises from a low of 15 per cent at five years of age to a peak of 33 per cent at 10 years, decreasing to 10 per cent at 18 years. [Malone and Massler, p. 199]

In comparing the age trend for severity of nailbiting with the age trend for number of fingers bitten (definite or indefinite nailbiters), Malone and Massler (1952) commented: "The age trend in the severe nailbiting group exactly duplicates the trend of the total group (per cent of children biting) and also the trend of the definite (10) fingernail biters" (p. 199). This trend indicated to Malone and Massler (1952) that children who severely bit all 10 fingernails "markedly influence[d] the trend for the total group" (p. 199). These children were identified as the true fingernail biters. Figure 9 represents a portion of a graph from Malone and Massler, depicting age trends for the number of fingernails bitten and the severity of fingernail biting. To reduce the amount of information charted, the trend for the non-nailbiters has been deleted.

Analysis of the data in the Malone and Massler research revealed that the differences in the number of boys and girls aged 5 to 10 years who bit their fingernails were not statistically significant. The differences, however, between the number of boys and girls who bit their fingernails from ages 10 to 18 were statistically significant. Generally, 10% fewer girls than boys in this age group bit their nails. The number of female nailbiters among the total group of children in the survey decreased "sharply at the age of nine years" (p. 194) and continued

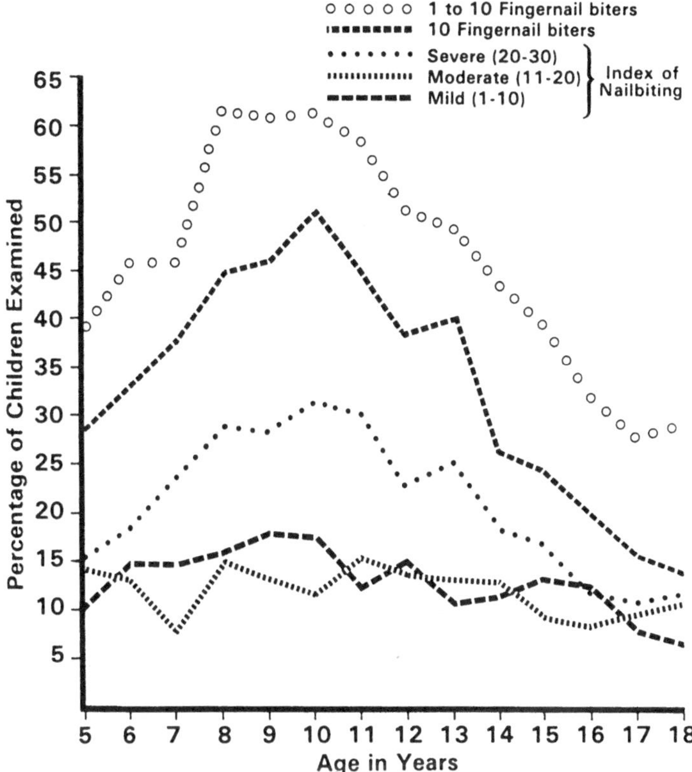

Figure 9 Graph showing age trends in fingernail biting according to number of fingernails bitten (1-10, 10) and severity of nailbiting (mild, moderate, and severe). Adapted from "Index of Nailbiting in Children," by A. J. Malone and M. Massler, *Journal of Abnormal and Social Psychology*, 1952, *47*, 193-202. Copyright by the American Psychological Association; reprinted with permission.

to decrease thereafter. A significant decrease in the number of male nailbiters was indicated at 11 years of age, with the numbers subsequently declining up to age 18. For the definite nailbiters, Massler and Malone found that "sex differences begin even earlier, at about eight years of age . . . . Girls begin to stop biting their fingernails at nine years of age, boys about one year later" (pp. 195-197). Among the small group of indefinite nailbiters, there appeared to be no significant sex differences at any age level from 5 to 18 years of age. The sex differences for the entire group of nailbiters, for the definite nailbiters, and for the indefinite nailbiters are illustrated in Figure 10.

Several age and sex trends of fingernail biting were identified by

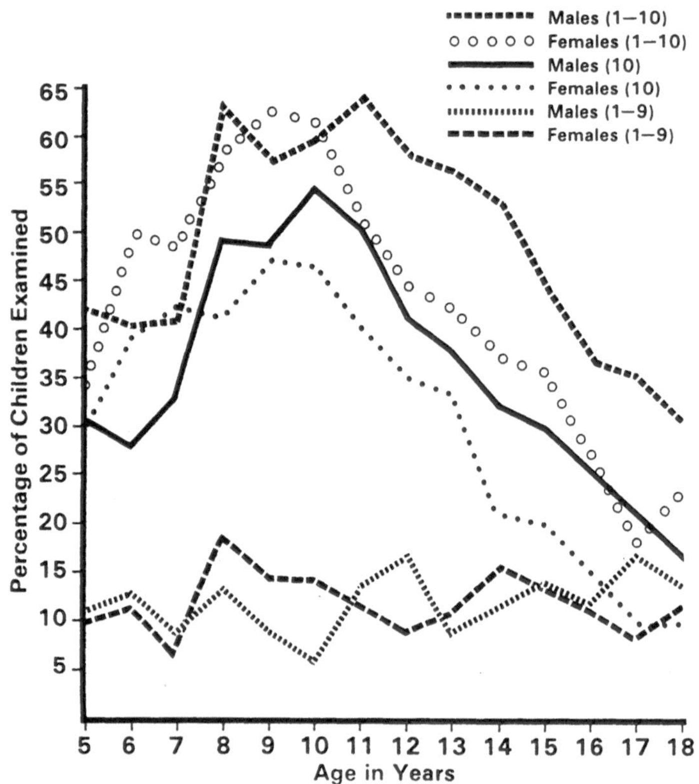

Figure 10 Sex differences in the number of fingernails bitten. Adapted from "Index of Nailbiting in Children," by A. J. Malone and M. Massler, *Journal of Abnormal and Social Psychology*, 1952, *47*, 193-202. Copyright by the American Psychological Association; reprinted with permission.

Wechsler (1931). He found that nailbiting did not occur under the age of three (p. 203), that it showed a gradual increase in prevalence up to age 6, and that the percentage of nailbiters then remained constant until age 12 in girls and age 14 for boys. At these ages, a sudden increase was noted for a period of 2 years and then a decline.

Illingworth (1964) concurred with the commonly found trend that nailbiting rarely occurs before the age of 3, but he interestingly commented that "the youngest nail-biter seen by . . . [him] was 18 months old" (p. 50).

In another early investigation, Koch (1935) studied 11 classes of mannerisms "frequently referred to as 'nervous habits' " (p. 140). A segment of Koch's investigation reported on the type and frequency of mannerisms exhibited by 21 boys and 25 girls of nursery-school age. This discussion will be limited to the two categories of mannerisms that are most pertinent to the present study: (a) the digital mannerism, which involved "playing with the fingers" and (b) the oral mannerisms of "sucking, biting, or chewing on things not intended for consumption" (p. 140). Although nailbiting is not specifically mentioned in the second category of activities, the findings related to this grouping of behaviors could have relevant implications for nailbiting behavior. Sex differences for the digital and oral mannerisms were not expected, yet were noted in finger play. Koch believed that the finding that finger play was more frequent among girls than boys was significant because "there are no obvious digital differences between the sexes" (p. 144). Table 4 illustrates a portion of the data from Koch relevant to sex differences in digital and oral mannerisms.

Birch (1955) found in his sample of 4,223 schoolchildren that significantly more boys than girls were nailbiters. The percentages of nailbiters among the schoolchildren showed a gradual increase up to age 8 and then remained fairly constant to age 14, after which a decline was evident. No marked peak periods were noted for either sex at any age level, with the exception of 12-year-old boys. The incidence of nailbiting for boys in this age group was "significantly higher than the percentage found for the whole male population" (Birch, p. 125). It was found that between the ages of 7 and 15 years a greater percentage of boys than girls bit their fingernails. For most age levels, however, the difference was not statistically significant. Another noticeable trend, although not significant, was the greater occurrence

Table 4 Sex Differences in Mean Number of Mannerisms for an Individual

	Boy		*Girl*		
Mannerism	*Mean*	*σ Dist.*	*Mean*	*σ Dist.*	*Critical ratio*
Oral	104.65	32.85	101.50	41.20	+ .29
Digital	57.25	14.75	65.10	16.75	−1.69

Adapted from "An Analysis of Certain Forms of So-called 'Nervous Habits' in Young Children," by H. L. Koch, *Journal of Genetic Psychology*, 1935, *46*, 139-170. Copyright by the Journal Press and reprinted with permission.

of biting among boys between the ages of 5 and 7 than among the girls in this same age group. The prevalence of nailbiting and the sex and age trends are illustrated in Figures 11 and 12.

Macfarlane et al. (1954) found that among the normal children in their longitudinal study of children's behavioral problems, the frequency of nailbiting rises in both boys and girls to reach its peak at late pubescence, with the girls showing consistently more nailbiting than boys until year 14 (pp. 94-95). The beginning age varied as did the number of years that the nailbiting persisted. Some children bit their nails at only one age level, whereas others bit at several age levels.

On the basis of clinical work, Bevans (1945) concluded that more boys than girls bite their fingernails (p. 58), but reported that she was unable to provide a rationale for this finding. Viets (1931) found that among her group of 75 nailbiters there was "a slight tendency for the habit to be more prevalent among the boys who were nine to eleven years old and among the girls who were over eleven" (p. 131).

Hill (1946) studied the prevalence of nailbiting among naval and marine enlisted personnel who were evacuated from the battle area to a hospital in the U.S. because of nervous conditions. From among 223 routine admissions, 100 of the men were nailbiters, which con-

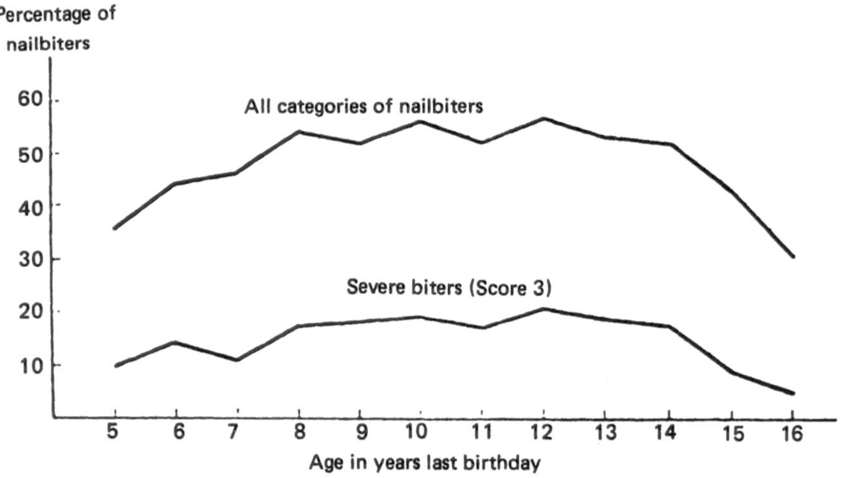

Figure 11 Percentage distribution of nail-biters (boys and girls together). From "The Incidence of Nail-biting Among School Children," by L. B. Birch, *British Journal of Educational Psychology*, 1955, *25*, 123-128. Copyright by the British Journal of Educational Psychology; reprinted with permission.

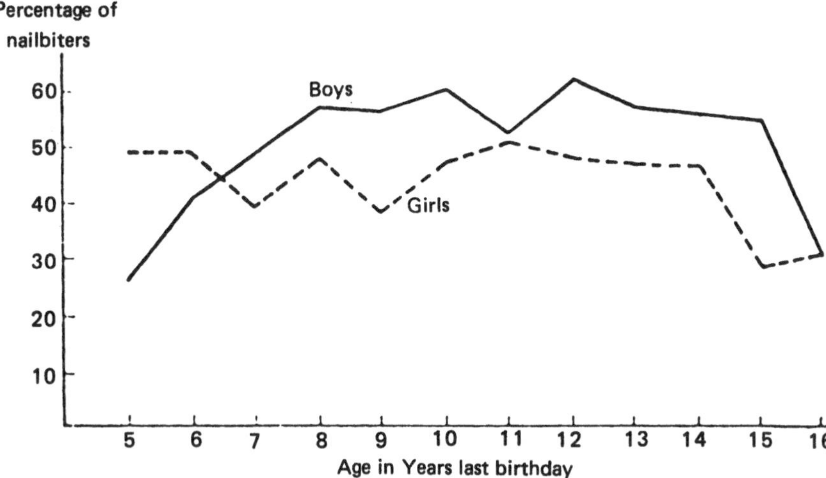

Figure 12 Percentage distribution of nail-biters (boys and girls separately). From "The Incidence of Nail-biting Among School Children," by L. B. Birch, *British Journal of Educational Psychology*, 1955, *25*, 123-128. Copyright by the British Journal of Educational Psychology; reprinted with permission.

stituted 45% of the sample. In addition, Hill found that half the nail-biters "bit their nails periodically or continuously since their earliest recollections" (p. 185). He compared this incidence of nailbiting to the incidence among a group of 1,571 naval male enlisted personnel who "had no sick list admissions because of nervousness" and found that only 6% were nailbiters (p. 187). Of the 100 cases of nailbiters among this group "more than half bit their nails as long as they could recall" (p. 187).

A preliminary questionnaire given to 1,077 college students (Coleman and McCalley, 1948a) revealed that approximately the same number of males and females were current nailbiters: 29.3% of the males and 19.3% of the females. In addition, "22.8 per cent of the males and 35.2 per cent of the females once bit their nails but have ceased" (p. 518). Table 5 illustrates the ages at which the former nail-biters in the Coleman and McCalley (1948a) study began and stopped nailbiting. These trends appear to indicate that the females generally began and ceased nailbiting at earlier ages than the males.

McNamara (1972) reported that sex differences were revealed in his study on self-monitoring techniques for the treatment of nailbiting among male and female college students. Analyses indicated that the

Table 5 Modal Age Ranges at Which Former Nailbiters Began and Stopped Biting Their Fingernails

	Began nailbiting	*Ceased nailbiting*
Males	5-12 yrs.	12-16 yrs.
Females	4-8 yrs.	10-14 yrs.

Adapted from "Nail-biting Among College Students," by J. C. Coleman and J. E. McCalley, *Journal of Abnormal and Social Psychology*, 1948, *43*, 517-525. Copyright by the American Psychological Association and reprinted with permission.

sexes differed in nail length; males had "significantly longer finger nails than did females at Week 2 . . . and at Week 4" (p. 193).

In cases of acute anxiety, Rushforth (1951) asserted that nailbiting "affects children and adults of all ages and of both sexes" (p. 192). Rushforth claimed that although there is a tendency to outgrow nailbiting, it is a frequently occurring symptom in anxious adults.

The prevalence of nailbiting among mentally retarded, mentally ill, and normal Britons was examined by Ballinger (1970). He found no statistically significant differences in prevalence among the groups except for 50- to 59-year-old mentally ill patients. For this group, the prevalence was significantly lower than for the same age group in the normal population. Psychiatric patients showed a peak prevalence (26.8%) between the ages of 30 and 39, whereas the peak prevalence in normals (35.2%) and mental defectives (28.4%) was between the ages of 10 and 19. A progressive decline in nailbiting was indicated after the age of 40 in all three groups. A portion of the data from Ballinger pertaining to age-group prevalence of nailbiting is summarized in Table 6.

A study by Michaels and Goodman (1934) contained a review of a number of published reports on the prevalence of various childhood behavioral problems (see Table 7). Their table has been modified to reveal only the prevalence of nailbiting behavior in various populations. In addition, I have attempted to update the table by adding the prevalence data obtained from studies published since 1934.

Table 6 Prevalence of Nailbiting Among Normals, Mental Defectives, and Psychiatric Patients

	Nailbiters		*Peak prevalence of nailbiting*		
Group	*Total* N^a	*Percent*	*Age Group*	*Total N*	*Percent*
Normal	832	23.1	10-19 yrs.	233	35.2
Mentally defective	626	20.1	10-19 yrs.	102	28.4
Mentally ill	584	7.4	30-39 yrs.	41	26.8

From "The Prevalence of Nail-Biting in Normal and Abnormal Populations," by B. R. Ballinger, *British Journal of Psychiatry*, 1970, *117*, 445-446. Copyright by the Royal College of Psychiatrists and reprinted with permission.

[a]Total N refers to the total number of subjects in all age ranges from 0-9 years to 70+ years for each of the three groups.

PERSONALITY CHARACTERISTICS

Using a standard set of 15 stimuli, Koch (1935) examined the relationship between mannerism counts and skin resistance measures by the galvanic skin response. About half of the stimuli were assumed to be pleasant, e.g., praising or kissing the child, showing a candy rabbit or some cookies; the remaining half were considered to be unpleasant, e.g., threatening with a rubber band or small gun. The stimuli were administered on two occasions, separated by periods of time ranging from a week to a month. Koch's findings revealed no significant correlations between the skin resistance measures and the occurrence of most mannerisms. With regard to finger play, however, Koch (1935) made the following comment:

> Focusing on the girls, we note what seems to be a dependable negative correlation between relative decrease in skin resistance and finger play. [p. 155]

Table 7 Percentage of Prevalence of Nailbiting, as Reported in Various Studies as Cited in Michaels and Goodman (1934)

Author	*Number and kind of cases*	*Percent*
Taylor (1922)	190 children	17.4
Bridges and Bridges (1926)	98 delinquent boys	50.0
	100 unselected boys	41.0
Foster and Stebbins (1929)	150 preschool children	6.0
Tilson (1929)	225 preschool children	6.2
Anderson (1930)	22-27 enuretic girls	68.0
	39-63 enuretic boys	41.0
Ward (1930)	100 only children	19.0
Ackerson (1931)	2,853 white boys	12.0
	1,739 white girls	18.0
	245 negro boys	10.0
	163 negro girls	6.0
Bowman and Raymond (1931)	50 schizophrenics	17.8
Wechsler (1931)	3,000 children, aged 1-17:	
	girls, 5-6 years	31.0
	boys, 5-6 years	27.1
	girls, 9-10 years	33.7
	boys, 9-10 years	38.5
	girls, 12-13 years	44.4
	boys, 12-13 years	35.0
	girls, 13-14 years	34.3
	boys, 13-14 years	43.6
Stevens (1932)	100 college freshman	31.0
	100 prison inmates	15.0
Michaels and Goodman (1934)	220 girls	57.1
	255 boys	45.7
	475 total (actually 440– no data for 35)	51.3
Billig (1941)	ward for behavioral problem children:	25.0
	132 10th-grade girls	25.0
	130 10th-grade boys and girls (combined data)	20.0
	117 5th- and 6th-grade boys	58.8
	95 5th- and 6th-grade girls	60.0
	223 4th- to 6th-grade boys and girls (combined data)	39.9
	boys	36.3
	girls	41.1
Pennington and Mearin (1944)	2,297 white military personnel (17-48 years):	23.2
	1,144 white naval volunteers	22.9
	1,153 white naval draftees	23.5

Table 7 *(continued)*

Author	*Number and kind of cases*	*Percent*
Pennington and Mearin (1944, *continued*)	150 negro volunteers	23.1
Pennington (1945)	4,649 white male naval personnel:	
	938 17-year-olds	27.7
	1,108 18- to 20-year-olds	20.9
	391 21- to 23-year-olds	14.8
	323 24- to 26-year-olds	13.2
	350 27- to 29-year-olds	11.2
	272 30- to 32-year-olds	9.1
	188 33- to 35-year-olds	9.5
	79 36- to 37-year-olds	8.9
Pennington and Mearin (1944); Pennington (1945): data combined	6,946 white male naval personnel	21.5
Hill (1946)	223 male naval and marine enlisted military personnel	45.0
Coleman and McCalley (1948a)	1,077 college undergraduate students[a]:	
	Present nailbiters	
	male	29.3
	female	19.3
	Former nailbiters	
	male	22.8
	female	35.2
Woodward and Mangus (1949)	543 first-graders	46.0
Malone and Massler (1952)	4,587 schoolchildren (5-18 years of age)	41.0
Gedda (1953) (cited in Klackenberg, 1971)	7-year-old children (number unspecified)	7.0
Birch (1955)	4,223 children, aged 5-16:	51.0
	1,692 girls	46.0
	2,531 boys	54.0
Jonsson and Kalvesten (1964) [cited in Klackenberg, 1971]	7- to 16-year-old boys (number unspecified)	20.0
Ballinger (1970)	832 normals	23.1
	626 mental defectives	20.1
	584 psychiatric patients	7.4

Adapted from "Incidence and Intercorrelations of Enuresis and Other Neuropathic Traits in So-called Normal Children," by J. J. Michaels and S. E. Goodman, *American Journal of Orthopsychiatry*, 1934, *4*, 79-106. [Author has updated the table by adding prevalence data obtained from studies published since 1934.]

[a]N for males and N for females is not provided in article.

Koch interpreted this finding to mean that a tendency to indulge in finger play is positively associated with introversion. This conclusion was based on her interpretation of evidence relating decreases in skin resistance with introversion. Koch's data were among the earliest available on the relationship between finger play and introversion.

Viets (1931) attempted to determine the prevalence of introversion and extroversion in 75 nailbiting and 75 nonnailbiting children. Her findings, presented in Table 8, indicate that more nailbiters than nonnailbiters were extroverted and also that slightly more nailbiters were extroverted than introverted. These evaluations of the relationship between nailbiting and introversion-extroversion were made on the basis of subjective ratings, which Viets (1931) recognized as being "inaccurate and exceptionally liable to the vagaries of the judge's interpretation, but the results throw some doubt on the association of nail-biting with seclusiveness" (p. 138). Subjectivity is evident on the basis of some of the characteristics attributed to introverts; such as, "seclusiveness, egocentricity, day-dreaming, submissiveness, being a follower, sensitiveness, immaturity" (Viets, 1931, p. 138). Children showing traits of "aggressiveness, independence, braggadocio, and leadership" (p. 138) were classified as being extroverted. The possible inaccuracy of this impressionistic information constituted Viets' first cautionary remark regarding her findings. Her second comment was related to the inconsistency between the nailbiting-extroversion relationship and indications of an interest in individual activities by two-thirds of the nailbiters. Viets (1931) made the following statement with regard to this inconsistency: "It might be expected that they [nailbiters] would be interested in group activities of a rather stren-

Table 8 Personality Types

Personality type	*Nailbiters*	*Control*
Normal	17	18
Introverted	28	36
Extroverted	30	21
Total	75	75

From "An Inquiry into the Significance of Nail-Biting," by L.. E. Viets, *Smith College Studies in Social Work*, 1931, *2*, 128-145. Copyright by Smith College of Social Work and reprinted with permission.

uous active type" (p. 137). Still another unexpected finding was that 35 of the 49 nailbiters for whom information was available had "few or no friends" (p. 137).

On the basis of the information in the Viets article, it appears that Viets' expectation was that fewer nailbiters would report that they had "few or no friends" than would report that they had many friends. Her expectation seemed to be based on her finding that there were more extroverted nailbiters than introverted nailbiters in her study and on her premise that extroverts would be interested in group activities and hence would have many friends.

In his study of 300 10th-grade boys and girls, Billig's (1941) results revealed that "64 per cent of the nail-biters, 47 per cent of the non-nail-biters, and 31 per cent of the former nail-biters exceeded the fiftieth (normal) percentile on the Bernreuter neurotic scale (B1-N) of the *Personality Inventory*" (p. 209). The nonnailbiting group appeared to be the "most normal of the three" (Billig, 1941, p. 191). In his summary of these findings, Billig reported that "the nail-biters were . . . more neurotic than either of the other two categories. . . the former nail-biters . . . were less neurotic than the non-nail-biters" (p. 192).

Nailbiting behavior was described by Jenkins (1973) within the context of a Type I personality. According to Jenkins:

> In Type I we see an individual who has an excessive development of the shell of inhibition. As a result of this the primitive impulses are denied adequate expression. Tension mounts within the personality and strong pressures develop in the struggle between the primitive impulses and the repressive forces. This individual is chronically in a state of internal conflict. Here we have the over-inhibited individual likely to react to these internal conflicts by developing terror dreams or anxiety attacks, or by developing physical symptoms of illness through conversion hysteria, or to defend himself from them by compulsive rituals. We do not, as a rule, see such well-developed neurotic symptoms in the child, but we see the milder over-inhibited symptoms of shyness, seclusiveness, fears, clinging, tics, sleep disturbances, nail biting, and other common evidences of tension and anxiety with which the child guidance worker is familiar. The essential

> points are to recognize that the person with severe internal conflict is, as a rule, the over-inhibited individual. [p. 29]

Coleman and McCalley (1948a) compared the college students in their control and experimental groups on the basis of scores on the neuroticism and extroversion-introversion scales of the Bernreuter Personality Inventory. Differences between the male nailbiters and male nonnailbiters were not statistically significant although "male nail-biters tended toward higher neurotic scores than male non-nail-biters" (p. 520). The male nailbiters also exhibited "a trend toward higher introversion scores than their non-nail-biting controls" (p. 520) but, as with the neuroticism scores, the difference was not significant. The summary of scores presented in Coleman and McCalley's study (1948a) appeared to indicate that, with statistically significant differences on both scales (significant above the 1% level), the female nailbiters were more introverted and more neurotic than the female nonnailbiters. The experimental groups (male and female) scored around the 50th percentile on both scales of the Bernreuter Personality Inventory, while the scores of the control groups were around the 37th percentile. Hence, Coleman and McCalley (1948a) commented:

> Interpreting the meaning of the obtained Bernreuter percentile scores of our experimental and control groups is a difficult task. If we accept the Bernreuter norms as valid, it must mean two things as regards our study: (1) that nail-biters are not neurotic or introverted in comparison with other college populations, and (2) that non-nail-biters are better adjusted than the average college population, that is, they are less introverted and less neurotic. It would also be possible to ignore the established Bernreuter norms, in which case we might say that, in comparison with non-nail-biters, nail-biters are more likely to have traits of neuroticism and introversion. This generalization is also true in the light of the first condition, accepting the norms, but is not so evident if we state our results from testing the experimental groups in percentile ranks without stating those of the control groups. However, it would appear desirable to use control groups and not rely entirely upon the standardized norms. Even if we accept their validity, the exclusive use of standardized norms

> without the benefit of control groups might obscure some of the most significant findings in such a study. [p. 522]

In attempting to explain why a significant difference in neuroticism was found between female nailbiters and female nonnailbiters, but not between male nailbiters and male nonnailbiters, Coleman and McCalley (1948a) attributed this partially to the "greater social pressure exerted on females to cease the nailbiting habit" (p. 522). In elaborating on this rationale, they commented that women continue to bite their nails despite social pressure to stop, which may be indicative of their need for this "tension-releasing mechanism" (p. 522). As Coleman and McCalley (1948a) stated: "It seems possible then that they may be under more tension and anxiety and hence would test on the Bernreuter scale as more "neurotic" than the nail-biting men" (p. 522). The following interpretation was offered by Coleman and McCalley (1948a) for their finding that the female nail-biters obtained significantly higher introversion scores than the female nonnailbiters: "Since ugly nails are less desirable socially than well-groomed hands, the female who bites her nails must withdraw herself from some areas of contact with society, and hence tends to become more introverted. Also it is possible that only the more introverted female nail-biters tend to continue the habit under social duress" (p. 522).

INTELLIGENCE FACTORS

Billig (1941) found in his study of 300 10th-grade pupils of both sexes that the group of former nailbiters had a mean IQ of 103.51, whereas the mean IQ of the nailbiters was 97.76. Those that never bit their nails had a mean IQ of 99.94, "which is essentially the same as the theoretical mean for intelligence at large" (Billig, 1941, p. 191). Intelligence was assessed by means of the Stanford Revision (1916) of the Binet-Simon tests.

In noting the 5.75 point-difference between the mean IQs of the former nailbiters and the present nailbiters, Billig (1941) suggested:

> Intelligence may at least facilitate the desisting of nail-biting. Individuals with higher than average intelligence possess more than average insight. These former nail-biters were apparently more

> successful with their respective problems than those still displaying nail-biting activity during their fifteenth year. This additional insight which the former nail-biters displayed may be a concomitant of their greater intelligence. [p. 191]

In Viets' (1931) research, intelligence ratings were based largely on the 1916 Stanford-Binet test. Upon comparing the nailbiting group with the nonnailbiting group, Viets concluded that "intelligence was not a factor associated with nail-biting" (p. 132).

Within a group of mentally retarded individuals, Ballinger (1970) found that the prevalence of nailbiting for individuals in the 0-19 IQ range was significantly lower than the prevalence for the other mental defectives. For those in the 68-and-above range of IQ, the occurrence of nailbiting was significantly higher than for those in the 0-68 range (Ballinger, 1970).

SITUATIONAL FACTORS

In analyzing responses to the question, "Do you bite your nails when you are working or playing at your hobby?," Billig (1941) found that female nailbiters in the children's ward of a hospital in the U. S. "very seldom bit their nails while occupied with their hobby" (p. 166). This finding was reported by Billig (1941) to have been substantiated by the observations of occupational supervisors.

Billig (1941) obtained data relating nailbiting to various leisure-time activities. Various types of entertainment were named and 10 female nailbiters at the 10th-grade level were asked to raise their hands when one was named in which they consistently bit their nails. The number of hands raised was tabulated for each form of entertainment. Table 9 summarizes the responses of the 10 nailbiters in the study. All of the 10 girls said motion pictures were provocative, eight said games, and six said stories, with other forms of entertainment having less stimulus value, as indicated by their rank in Table 9.

Billig (1941) found agreement between female nailbiters and female nonnailbiters concerning the attributes of nailbiters. He asked a group of 50 nonnailbiters and 10 nailbiters of the 10th grade to list "three facts which they believed to be true . . . of nail-biters" (p. 170). A checklist of possible characteristics was not provided in advance

Table 9 Stimulus Value of Entertainment to Nailbiters Among Tenth-Grade Girls (Ten Cases)

Rank	*Entertainment*	*Frequency*
1	Motion Pictures	10
2	Games	8
3	Stories	6
4	Dances	4
5	Daydreaming	3
6	Parties	2
7	Picnics	1
8	Dates with Boys	1

From "Finger Nail-Biting: Its Incipiency, Incidence, and Amelioration," by A. L. Billig, *Genetic Psychology Monographs*, 1941, *24*, 123-218. Copyright by the Journal Press and reprinted with permission.

and opinions mentioned only once were not included in the summary of the responses. The typical responses made by the girls are summarized in Table 10 in order of the frequency of their occurrence. Billig reported that the girls of both groups appeared to believe that nervousness was the cause of nailbiting. He commented:

> They did not realize that the term "nervousness" is a descriptive term and could not possibly be the causal factor. . . . In these interviews, the pupils were asked to explain what this "nervousness" was. They would usually say, "*I cannot explain, I am just nervous, I was always this way.*" [Billig, 1941, p. 172]

The students' elaborations on the second most frequently cited response, "excitement," revealed that "the 'excitement' cited by the pupils seems to be of two origins: (a) being teased (anger), or (b) a perceived crisis (fear)" (Billig, 1941, p. 173). The girls' elaborations on the characteristic, "it occurs when one is idle," indicated that they actually meant that they were not able to do what they would like to be doing. According to Billig (1941), the typical explanation of this response amounted to:

> comparing what they were doing with what they would have liked to be doing. In these situations the things they were required to do were done automatically and to them this did not

Table 10 Reported Facts Believed Concerning Nailbiters: Girls

Believed facts	*Frequency*
They are nervous	42
They are excited	24
It is a habit	20
They are hungry	13
It occurs when one is idle	10
They do it because of fear	9
Because they are worried	8
They are unaware of doing it	6
They are not healthy	6
They are high-tempered	5
They enjoy it	4
They do it when they are thinking	4
They are irritable	3
They lack control of their feelings	2
It is due to conditions in the home	2
Because they cannot chew gum	2
They do not eat much	2

From "Finger Nail-Biting: Its Incipiency, Incidence, and Amelioration," by A. L. Billig, *Genetic Psychology Monographs*, 1941, *24*, 123-218. Copyright by the Journal Press and reprinted with permission.

> really seem to be "doing." Only doing what they would like to do would be "real doing." [pp. 172-173]

This finding seems to be consistent with those reported by Billig in another segment of his 1941 study. Presumably, the female nailbiters in the children's hospital ward who reported that they seldom bit their nails when involved in their hobbies were doing what they wished; hence, the reduced frequency of nailbiting in these instances.

In summary, Billig (1941) found that the three most frequently cited facts believed by 10th-grade girls to be true of nailbiters were "nervousness," "excitement," and the fact that it is a "habit" (p. 171). There appears to be some consensus between these findings and the reports by nailbiters in various studies investigating the actual circumstances associated with nailbiting behavior. For example, elements of nervousness, excitement, idleness, and the "habit" characteristic were evident in the findings of many researchers (Birch, 1955; Coleman and McCalley, 1948a; Hill, 1946; Koch, 1935; Malone and Massler, 1952; Pennington and Mearin, 1944).

In the Malone and Massler study (1952), the situations in which most of the children reported that they bit their fingernails were those which "made them nervous (watching exciting movies, during school examinations, radio and television programs, family quarrels, and sports events)" (p. 201). Boredom, which was attributed to "enforced inactivity in school" (p. 201), reportedly accounted for biting among 25% of the nailbiters. No reason for biting was given by 16% of the nailbiters. The 1,077 college students who completed a preliminary questionnaire for Coleman and McCalley (1948a) were categorized into three distinct groups: present nailbiters, former nailbiters, and nonnailbiters. The present nailbiters gave various reasons for their nailbiting behavior, as indicated by Coleman and McCalley (1948a):

> (1) The desire to keep busy and to use up what seemed to the subject to be excess energy, (2) anxiety and stress connected with situations such as final examinations, athletic events, social events, and various personal problems, (3) unconsciously and/or as a habit with no explanation. Almost all agreed that, the greater the tension, the more frequent the nail-biting. [p. 519]

In investigating the circumstances under which nailbiting most frequently occurred, Hill (1946) obtained information from 100 nailbiters who were among 223 military enlistees admitted to hospital because of nervous conditions. Hill found evidence of primarily three characteristic situations associated with nailbiting behavior. The first set of circumstances were "tense, emotional situations," as reflected in statements made by the nailbiters: " 'when I am mad and can't do anything about it'; when observing movies of murder and war; and in combat, after it, or while thinking of it" (Hill, p. 185). The second set of circumstances were associated with enforced inactivity. According to Hill, "a second frequent occasion for nail biting was during periods of inactivity enforced by others or themselves. A desired result was to aid in concentrating attention, as 'to clear my mind when about to fight,' and 'to make decisions' " (p. 185). A third set of responses suggested that the nailbiter had limited awareness of the circumstances surrounding his episodes of nailbiting. For example:

> A casual explanation of nail biting was described as "just catch myself doing it, not thinking." Here there was usually the interpolation, "ashamed of doing it," or "I know better." These addenda were given voluntarily by those whose nail biting started in childhood. Other explanations were, "don't know," and "just a habit, like smoking." [Hill, 1946, p. 185]

Pennington and Mearin (1944) studied the behavior of nailbiting among 2,297 recruits in attempting to determine the circumstances most frequently associated with nailbiting. Each recruit was asked the following two questions: "(1) Under what circumstances do you bite your nails the most? (2) Why do you bite them?" (p. 629). Of the 2,297 men examined, 533 (23.2%) were nailbiters. Thus, "one man in 4.31 selectees exhibited evidence of the habit [nailbiting]" (Pennington and Mearin, 1944, p. 629). The answers to these two questions for 508 out of 533 recruits "addicted in any degree to nailbiting" (p. 630) were tabulated according to various nailbiting-associated circumstances. The data presented in Table 11 are adapted from Pennington and Mearin, 1944.

Billig (1941) attempted to determine which of a number of basic conditions were believed to be most responsible for evoking the

Table 11 Classified Responses to Circumstances Associated with Nailbiting

Response class	*Frequency*
At the movies	151
I don't (denial)	32
Nothing to do	69
Waiting around	17
To cut them	96
When I'm upset	46
I'm quitting	24
I don't know when	51
Miscellaneous	22

Adapted from "The Frequency and Significance of a Movement Mannerism for the Military Psychologist," by L. A. Pennington and R. J. Mearin, *American Journal of Psychiatry*, 1944, *100*, 628-632.

behavior of nailbiting. Twenty-six nailbiters of the 10th grade, most of whom were girls, were asked to indicate which of the following four conditions contributed most to their nailbiting activity: (a) Delay in time between stimulus and response (suspense); (b) making discrimination too subtle; (c) overstraining; and (d) two opposite activities (as something very pleasant and very disagreeable) at the same time (Billig, 1941, p. 171). The choices made by the nailbiters from the four stimulus situations are listed in Table 12.

Razran (cited in Billig, 1941) held the opinion that of the four stimulus conditions, the most prepotent for evoking nailbiting behavior was the situation of "two opposite activities" (p. 173). However, information obtained and reported in Table 12 indicates that "suspense," or delay between stimulus and response was the most prepotent. Billig stressed that the data in Table 12 apply mainly to adolescent girls. Results may be quite different for males and for different age groups.

According to Shahovitch (1945), the occurrence of nailbiting in children is attributed to the presence of one or more stimulus conditions. One of these conditions is the moving about of families, which brings the child into an endless number of new situations. Another is the excessive emotional stimulation provided by scenes of violence in television programs. Even the stimulating effects of "the drink containing caffeine" (p. 303) was believed by Shahovitch (1945) to predispose an individual to fingernail biting. A fourth condition relates

Table 12 Prepotent Stimulus Situations Eliciting Nailbiting: Both Sexes

Stimulus situation	*Frequency*
Suspense	19
Discrimination too subtle	2
Overstraining	2
Two opposite activities	3
Total	26

From "Finger Nail-biting: Its Incipiency, Incidence, and Amelioration," by A. L. Billig, *Genetic Psychology Monographs*, 1941, *24*, 123-218. Copyright by the Journal Press and reprinted with permission.

to the child's having too few household responsibilities and therefore little occupation for his hands.

In investigating the relationship between the type of activity and display of mannerisms, Koch (1935) observed children in situations that permitted them varying degrees of freedom. One hundred ½-minute time samples were obtained on each child's behavior as observed during each of four kinds of activities: free play indoors, free play outdoors, controlled play indoors, and routines such as washing, dressing, and undressing. Koch's findings pertaining to the type of activity and the digital and oral mannerisms are summarized in Table 13. *Digital mannerism* refers to "playing with the fingers"; *oral mannerisms* refer to "sucking, biting, or chewing on things not intended for consumption" (p. 140). These data have been extracted from a more detailed table in Koch, 1935.

Koch's finding that "mannerisms generally occur with greater frequency in indoor play than outdoor, and in controlled play than in free" (p. 148) concurred with her view that restraint favors mannerisms. She offered three distinct explanations for the generally greater frequency of bodily directed mannerisms during restriction of activities:

> [1.] Stimuli set up impulses which must find a motor outlet; and if they cannot effect this in purposeful acts involving the body grossly, they will do so in more or less irrelevant activity. . . .
>
> [2.] Offences against the ego which occasion emotional upsets occur more often in controlled play than in the other activities. . . .

Table 13 Relationship Between Type of Mannerisms and Degree of Freedom in Activity

	Mean Number of Mannerisms			
Mannerism	*Free play indoors*	*Free play outdoors*	*Routines*	*Controlled play indoors*
Digital	14.63	10.70	9.57	27.72
Oral	26.04	25.66	21.18	30.96

Adapted from "An Analysis of Certain Forms of So-Called 'Nervous Habits' in Young Children," by H. L. Koch, *Journal of Genetic Psychology*, 1935, *46*, 139-170. Copyright by the Journal Press and reprinted with permission.

> [3.] Attention is less dynamically held by the games dictated by the teacher and thus is focused more readily upon minor body irritations. [pp. 145-147]

The tendency to play alone was found by Koch to be negatively correlated with the digital and oral mannerisms. In her interpretation of this finding, Koch reasoned that when playing alone many children become absorbed in an activity, which in turn provides little occasion for finger play and oral mannerisms. A tendency toward watching others is positively correlated with a proneness to finger manipulation.

Birch (1955) conducted a survey of 4,223 schoolchildren aged 5 to 16 years. Of the 473 nailbiters in the 8- to 10-year old range, 54% reported that they either were unaware of their nailbiting behavior or had no preference for the time or place of biting; 23% said they bit while watching television or a movie; 8% when reading; 11% when concentrating on a school subject; 5% when they were bored; 2% when worried. About half the group who reported biting when bored said that they bit their nails when in bed.

During interviews with a small number of female nailbiters in the children's ward of a state hospital in the U. S., Billig (1941) reported that most of these nailbiters claimed that they were unaware of the act of nailbiting. This conclusion was based on the responses to the question, "Do you know when you are biting them [your fingernails]?" (p. 165). Verbatim samples of the girls' responses were not provided, but most answers to the question, "Why do you think you bite your nails?" were, according to Billig, "the type that would be expected from adults. The patients probably heard these answers, at some time or another, and were merely repeating them" (p. 166). In a regular school setting, Billig (1941) found that 81 of the 89 nailbiters in grades 4, 5, and 6, varying in age from 8 to 15, reported that they were aware of the act of nailbiting. This indicated that 91% knew they were biting their nails. "Tenth grade students also said they were aware of indulging" (Billig, 1941, p. 207).

Additional comments concerning awareness of nailbiting are made in other works (Adesso, Vargas, and Siddall, 1979; Azrin and Nunn, 1977; Perkins and Perkins, 1976; Vargas and Adesso, 1976) and occur in this monograph within the context of treatment procedures for nailbiting (see Chapter 5).

FAMILY VARIABLES

One of the variables investigated in the Viets (1931) study was family size. The data revealed several trends:

1. In two-child families, there were as many nailbiters as non-nailbiters.
2. Among two-child families, the nailbiters were predominantly girls, whereas in three- and four-child families, they were predominantly boys.
3. The greatest difference in the number of nailbiters and non-nailbiters occurred in four-child families, where the ratio was 14 nailbiters to 6 nonnailbiters.

As indicated by Viets, these findings were not statistically significant.

Koch (1935) investigated the relationship between a number of home conditions and mannerism frequency. Included among these movement mannerisms were the digital and oral mannerisms previously defined. Number of playmates was found to be positively correlated with oral mannerisms for boys and girls (+.313) and with the digital mannerism for boys (+.187). These findings seem to be inconsistent, however, with three other correlations: (a) a negative correlation between the number of siblings/persons in the household and oral mannerisms for boys and girls together (- .038/- .164); (b) a very low positive correlation between the number of sibling/persons in the household and the digital mannerism in boys (+.069/+.085); (c) a negative correlation between these two home conditions and the digital mannerism in girls (- .324/- .260). Koch (1935) postulated that "a large number of playmates may result in much competition and strain which in turn may provoke mannerisms or excess movements" (p. 151). She also found it difficult to "harmonize the findings relative to sibs and playmates" (p. 151). Table 14 contains a brief summary of the findings pertinent to the above discussion, as taken from Koch, 1935.

The relationship between a child's ordinal birth position and nailbiting behavior was researched by Viets. Although ordinal position has been "recognized as being highly important" (Viets, 1931, p. 141), the results of this study revealed that nailbiting does not appear to favor youngest, middle, oldest, or only-child ordinal positions. In Table 15, note how similarly the nailbiters and the control subjects were distributed with respect to ordinal position.

Table 14 Correlations Between Movement Mannerism Scores and Various Measures of Home Conditions

Mannerism	*No. of sibs*	*No. of playmates*	*No. in household*	*No. for a room in house*	*No. of residences since birth*
Oral (boys and girls)	-.038	+.313	-.164	-.107	-.093
Digital (boys)	+.069	+.187	+.085	-.273	+.169
Digital (girls)	-.324	-.406	-.260	-.252	+.232
Digital (total)	-.147	-.129	-.099	-.220	+.161

Adapted from "An Analysis of Certain Forms of So-called 'Nervous Habits' in Young Children," by H. L. Koch, *Journal of Genetic Psychology*, 1935, *46*, 139-170. Copyright by the Journal Press and reprinted with permission.

Table 15 Ordinal Position [and Nailbiting]

Ordinal position	*Boys*		*Girls*		*Total*	
	Nailbiters	*Control*	*Nailbiters*	*Control*	*Nailbiters*	*Control*
Youngest	9	13	9	7	18	20
Middle	15	15	7	6	22	21
Oldest	19	20	9	4	28	24
Only	3	5	4	5	7	10
Total	46	53	29	22	75	75

From "An Inquiry into the Significance of Nail-biting," by L. E. Viets, *Smith College Studies in Social Work*, 1931, *2*, 128-145. Copyright by Smith College School of Social Work and reprinted with permission.

From the available data for the normal children in the Berkeley Guidance Study, Macfarlane, Allen and Honzik (1954) found that from ages 1¾ to 13, the average number of first-born girls who were nailbiters was greater than the mean number of first-born boys, non-first-born girls, or non-first-born boys. Data from Macfarlane et al. (1954) pertinent to the incidence of nailbiting in first-born and non-first-born children are presented in Table 16. None of the differences between first-born and non-first-born was significant at either the 5% or 1% levels (Macfarlane et al., 1954).

Table 16 Percentage of Nailbiting Incidence Among First-Born and Non-first-born Children Aged 1¾ to 13 years

	Age in years												
Sib order	*1¾*	*3*	*4*	*5*	*6*	*7*	*8*	*9*	*10*	*11*	*12*	*13*	
	Total number												
First-born boys	24	19	18	13	14	14	14	15	15	12	8	10	
Non-first-born boys	32	30	27	26	20	21	18	20	12	15	15	14	
First-born girls	28	24	27	27	26	24	24	25	18	20	21	17	
Non-first-born girls	32	25	22	25	23	24	19	18	16	18	21	17	
	Percentage nailbiting												*Average*
First-born boys	4	5	11	8	21	29	7	13	13	33	12	30	15.5
Non-first-born boys	6	10	7	8	5	19	22	25	25	27	27	36	18.1
First-born girls	7	8	22	26	27	33	33	48	39	40	43	29	29.6
Non-first-born girls	0	12	5	8	13	21	11	17	25	39	19	24	16.2

Adapted from *A developmental study of behavior problems of normal children between twenty-one months and fourteen years*, by J. W. Macfarlane, L. Allen, and M. P. Honzik, Berkeley, Ca.: University of California Press, 1954. Copyright by the University of California Press and reprinted with permission.

RELATION TO OTHER BEHAVIORAL PROBLEMS

The incidence of behavior disorders among 475 boys and girls aged 6 to 19 was investigated by Michaels and Goodman (1934). They found that in their nailbiting group of 226 boys and girls, 57% showed one or more of four other behavioral problems, i.e., enuresis, thumb-sucking, speech impediments, and tantrums. These researchers found that 41% of the same nailbiting sample showed none of the other four problems. The difference between these two percentages was reported by Michaels and Goodman to be statistically significant, as were the differences in the percentages for enuresis and tantrums. These percentages are illustrated in Table 17, which has been adapted from a summary of findings presented in tabular form in the Michaels and Goodman study. One may conclude from the results of this study that a large percentage of children who bite their fingernails do not have the other behavioral problems of enuresis, thumb-sucking, speech impediments, or tantrums (41% in this sample). Although 57% of the nailbiters showed one or more of the other behavioral problems, Michaels and Goodman (1934) found that nailbiting entered "least significantly in its association with the constellation of the other four . . . [behavioral problems]" (p. 95). In other words, the presence of a conglomerate of four *other* behavioral problems was less likely to occur in nailbiters than in children exhibiting any one of the other behavioral problems. Perhaps another conclusion that can be drawn

Table 17 Percentage of Behavioral Problem Children Showing Presence or Absence of Other Problems

Problems	*One or more present*	*None of the other four problems present*
Enuresis	27	16
Thumb-sucking	30	25
Nailbiting	57	41
Speech impediments	24	20
Tantrums	16	7

Adapted from "Incidence and Intercorrelations of Enuresis and Other Neuropathic Traits in So-called Normal Children," by J. J. Michaels and S. E. Goodman, *American Journal of Orthopsychiatry*, 1934, *4*, 79-106. Copyright by the American Orthopsychiatric Association and reprinted with permission.

from these findings is that when nailbiting is observed in a child, it may be indicative of the presence of one or more other behavioral problems but not necessarily of the presence of a large conglomerate of difficulties.

Despite the common oral component of the nailbiting and thumb-sucking mannerisms, Bakwin and Bakwin (1968) stressed that they tend to favor very different psychological and physiological types: "Nail-biting . . . is most commonly seen in tense, excitable children, in contrast to thumb-sucking, which is more likely to occur in children who are outwardly calm and placid" (p. 462). Their thesis, although intuitively appealing, is not accompanied by a theoretical rationale or by supporting data.

Gibson (1971) maintained that "like thumb-sucking . . . [nailbiting] occurs in children who are unhappy or worried" (p. 121). Sarles and Heisler (1978) agreed on this point, noting that "others would define nailbiting as a variation of thumb sucking since this behavior is also typically seen during times of stress" (p. 591).

Richardson (cited in Viets, 1931), in discussing the nervous child, said: "Nail-biting differs from thumb sucking in that the former cannot be considered a normal act at any stage of development, whereas the latter is a persistence of something that is normal at one stage of the child's development" (p. 128). It has been often noted that the mannerism of nailbiting chronologically follows thumb-sucking (Sim and Finn, 1973). Illingworth (1964), however, rejected the notion "that nail-biting may result from condemnation of the thumb-sucking habit" and proposed that "both nail-biting and thumb-sucking are associated with a particular types of personality" (p. 51). He did not, however, identify this personality type.

According to Klackenberg (1971), the assumption that nailbiting is a substitute symptom for thumb-sucking is usually made on the basis of the following observation: "If the first report of the child nailbiting has been received in the same year as it stopped thumb-sucking, or the year after, a connection has been assumed possible" (p. 65). Any relation, however, between the cessation of thumb-sucking and the commencement of nailbiting was found by Klackenberg to be not statistically significant. In accordance with this conclusion, he stated:

> Of . . . 106 children reported as nailbiting, regardless of the degree of intensity, at some point between 2 and 8 years, there were only 12 whose abandonment of thumbsucking showed any conceivable chronological relation to the commencement of nailbiting. This proportion is within the limits of chance. [Klackenberg, 1971, p. 66]

In further elaborating on the question of mutual exclusiveness between nailbiting and thumb-sucking, Klackenberg (1971) stated that "nailbiting can begin while a child is still fingersucking" (p. 66).

Macfarlane et al. (1954) noted a decrease in the frequency of thumb-sucking with age and a reverse trend for nailbiting. Some children were thumb-suckers and nailbiters concurrently, but usually "they were not concurrent and the thumbsucking came first" (p. 96). Also, "there were thumbsuckers who never became nailbiters and there were nailbiters who, from 20 months on, at least, had not sucked their thumbs" (p. 96).

Bakwin (1971) empirically studied the relationship between nailbiting and finger-sucking behavior. The information contained in Table 18 for same-sex twins ranging in age from 6 to 18 indicated the absence of an oral trend or association between finger-sucking and nailbiting.

The relationship between nailbiting and behavioral problems such

Table 18 Comparison of Incidence of Nailbiting in All Twin Children and in Twin Children with Persistent Finger-sucking

	Nailbiting in all twin children		*Nailbiting in twin children with persistent finger-sucking*	
	No.	*Percent*	*No.*	*Percent*
Total	203	30	61	29
Boys	81	24	23	21
Girls	122	37	38	27

From "Nail-biting in Twins," by H. Bakwin, *Developmental Medicine and Child Neurology*, 1971, *13*, 304-307. Copyright by Spastics International Medical Publications and reprinted with permission.

as defiance, temper tantrums, and biting of playmates was investigated by Klackenberg (1971). The data for this study were extracted from the 1964 longitudinal Stockholm study by Jonsson and Kälvesten (cited in Klackenberg, 1971). The information about the children in the 1964 study has been provided by their mothers. For a child to be included in Klackenberg's persistent nailbiting group, nailbiting had to have been noted at 5 or more of 7 annual interviews between the ages of 2 and 8 years. Of the 212 children in the longitudinal study, 106 were nailbiters and of these, a group of 22 children were designated as persistent nailbiters.

In testing for a possible covariation of temper tantrums and nailbiting behavior, Klackenberg (1971) first determined whether or not children noted for temper tantrums were also persistent nailbiters. Children who were described by their mothers as being particularly temperamental during the interviews when they were 6, 7, and 8 years old were compared with the other children in the study. The result was a random distribution. Another test was made to determine whether or not children noted for daily temper tantrums at 4 and 5 years were nailbiters at ages 6, 7, and 8. Klackenberg (1971) reported that "the incidence was no more than coincidental" (p. 66). The majority of the 4- and 5-year-old children at follow-up between the ages of 6 and 8 years had a more restrained disposition, with "no notable increase in the frequency of nailbiting" (Klackenberg, 1971, p. 66). The interpretation given by Klackenberg to this trend in the follow-up data of the 4- and 5-year-old children was that:

> Temper tantrums are a typical age-related symptom. As they grow older, children generally seem able to channel their tempestuous feelings over disappointments into more socially acceptable forms than bodily expression. Presumably those around the child show less disapproval of nailbiting than of the child lying on the floor and thrashing with its feet. If the changes of temperament occurring between 6 and 8 years are an expression of self-control, it is clear that nailbiting does not serve as a vicarious outlet for the emotions to any significant extent. [p. 67]

In investigating whether or not a relationship existed between nailbiting and defiance, Klackenberg (1971) compared those children who were reported to be "most difficult at 2 of 3 interviews between

[ages] 6 and 8 years (classified as 'often or always defiant when corrected')" (p. 66) with the rest of the children. The result was that "the particularly defiant children included more members of the group of persistent nailbiters than can be attributed to chance" (pp. 66-67). The established covariation between nailbiting and defiance "was hardly coincidental," according to Klackenberg (p. 71). He stressed, however, that:

> The situations in which a child or adult bites his nails are not as a rule consciously related to defiance or aggression but are more often than not described as a means of releasing emotional tension (1) [Billig, 1941]. The reasons for this tension can vary considerably and bear no apparent relation to an aggressive frame of mind. The influence giving rise to a symptom and converting it into a habit may be forgotten and the release which the habit provides may then be used for other reasons and purposes. [p. 67]

Klackenberg cautioned that inhibited aggression, which may have been the original cause of the nailbiting, may no longer be the actual cause. Instead of functioning as a release for aggression, it may now serve as a tension-release. Unfortunately, he did not account for the change in function.

Klackenberg (1971) studied the relation of nailbiting to other forms of biting in 1½- to 5-year-olds, especially the habit of biting their siblings, playmates, and parents. The following trend was reported: "At 3 years, the figures for biting are 22%, at 4 years 15% and at 5 years 7%" (p. 68). In testing the covariation between persistent nailbiting and other forms of biting among these children, Klackenberg (1971) found that "it does not occur in the same individuals more than one might expect from coincidence" (p. 68). In discussing the implication of this finding, Klackenberg (1971) wrote that research needs to be directed toward the possible aggressive nature of nailbiting and its role as a substitute for aggressive biting. With respect to this issue, Klackenberg (1971) commented:

> Assuming that nailbiting is an aggressive symptom (directed against the child's own body), one might expect, theoretically speaking, to find a demonstrable relation between aggressive biting and nailbiting. Nailbiting rises in frequency at the same time

> as aggressive biting declines as a result of development or of the pressure exerted by those around the child. The extroverted act of aggression is then forced into other channels, in order that the child can attain the acceptance it seeks. Nailbiting might be interpreted as a reserve channel of this kind for venting emotions of an aggressive natur[e]. [pp. 68-69].

Klackenberg noted that biting habits, other than nailbiting, were prominent up to the age of 5. He referred to these habits as an "obviously aggressive symptom" and added that the aggressive component of these biting habits "becomes more prominent with increasing age" (p. 68). In qualifying this statement, Klackenberg (1971) commented that "at least, this behavior [biting] is interpreted as unfriendly by those who fall victim to it" (p. 68).

Further discussion of the aggressive component of biting focused on a comparison between parental reaction to nailbiting and to other forms of biting. With regard to the biting of sibling or playmates, Klackenberg (1971) indicated that the usual consequence of this response is punishment of various sorts such as "reproof or sending the child to bed or . . . corporal punishment" (p. 68). He stated that "there is a striking difference between this reaction [to biting] and the milder response to nailbiting" and noted that "preventive or diversionary measures are reported less often [for biting]" (p. 68).

A longitudinal study of behavioral problems of normal children revealed that for nailbiting, "no significant relationships to other problems were found before age 5" (Macfarlane et al., 1954, p. 95). At 12 years of age, however, an interesting pattern was evident between the boys and girls. Nonjealous and nonoversensitive girls bit their nails at this age, whereas jealous and oversensitive boys showed evidence of nailbiting. Macfarlane et al. (1954) indicated that they have "no explanation for the difference in sign in the correlations at age 12 for boys and girls on *jealousy and oversensitiveness*" (p. 95).

The children were categorized on the basis of a five-point coding scale, with each of the five-scale points accompanied by a descriptive statement. Several categories were indicative of problematic behavior while others represented nonproblematic behavior. For the sensitivity item, a coding of 1, 2, or 5 indicated oversensitive behavior and a coding of 3 or 4 represented nonoversensitive behavior. For the jealousy scale, a coding of 1, 2 or 3 indicated jealous behavior while code 4 or 5 indicated nonjealousy.

4

Theories on the Cause of Nailbiting

TENSION-NAILBITING ISSUE

The role of anxiety in the etiology of nailbiting has been documented in the literature. In commenting on the consensus of evidence concerning the relation of nailbiting to tense emotional situations, Massler and Malone (1950) stated that "the adage that persons under tension 'bite their nails' seems to be true" (p. 526). Tyron (cited in Pierce, 1975) acknowledged the possible tension-reducing function of nailbiting under conditions of boredom or anxiety. The nonsymptomatic nature of nailbiting is stressed in his statement, "the habit is often present in persons in whom there is no obvious emotional disturbance" (Tyron, cited in Pierce, 1975, p. 2126). Pierce also concurred with the tension-nailbiting hypothesis on the assumption that nailbiting is thought to be "the result of regression to oral satisfactions when the person is placed under the duress of tension or fatigue" (p. 2126).

Bowley provided an interesting illustration of a possible link between teacher-emitted censure, nagging, etc., and nailbiting behavior. In this respect, she wrote:

> I remember once being asked to call on a headmaster of a primary school to discuss this question of nail-biting. It appeared that in one particular class almost every child was a nail-biter!

> The common factor here was a particularly severe teacher who had reduced the class to a state of acute nervous tension. [Bowley, 1966, pp. 72-73]

Limited though Bowley's example may be, it is nonetheless one of the few published accounts that extends the tension-nailbiting issue to situations other than the child's home environment. If nailbiting is related to tension, it seems logical that tension-producing environments other than the home would be associated with nailbiting.

Although Massler and Malone (1950) referred to nailbiting among grade-school children as being normal, they stressed that the "unavoidable tensions of the average home and school environments" (p. 527) should be recognized and evaluated. This relates directly to their belief that "nailbiting is evidence of internal tensions" (Massler and Malone, p. 527). They added that a mild degree of nailbiting could be considered normal but cautioned that severe persistent nailbiting "must be significant and indicative of more than ordinary internal tensions" (p. 527). Kanner (1972) briefly mentioned two factors that affect the intensity of nailbiting. Specifically, "the intensity [of nailbiting] varies with the degree of tension and with the occasion" (p. 529). He cited some examples of the occasions on which boys and girls bite their nails:

> One boy practiced the habit only when watching others play ball. Another boy "got confused and bit his nails if he missed his lessons and the teacher kept him in to explain things to him." A little girl indulged mainly when she met strangers. Any excitement causes some youngsters to lose all self-control in this respect. [Kanner, 1972, pp. 529-530]

Langford (1972) held the following view about nailbiting:

> It is an expression of tenseness, being usually found in fidgety, overactive children. . . . Treatment should be directed at the child to relieve the causes of his tension. . . . Nagging and constantly calling the child's attention to his difficulty serve only to increase the existing tension. [p. 276]

One rather general conception that has been formulated concerning tension and nailbiting is that the child who bites his nails is an extremely nervous child. Griffith (cited in Viets, 1931), for instance, said "nail-biting is observed only in decidedly nervous children and may persist more or less during life unless vigorously treated" (p. 128).

Between 1940 and 1945 in the United States, Billig (1946) collected data on the incidence of nailbiting among 14- to 16-year-old students at the 10th-grade level. The incidence of nailbiting appeared consistent in samples taken at yearly intervals from 1940 to 1945, even though periods of "peace, war, and peace again" (p. 42) were encompassed in the time span. The proportion of nailbiters did not increase in a systematic way during this period of increased tension and anxiety. According to Billig (1946):

> It seems that marginal irritations set off nail-biting. The biting appears to serve as an ameliorative for such irritations. The serious tensions do not seem to be directly related to nail-biting but are manifested in other behavioral responses of a more complex organization, such as: dancing, talking, arguing, and fighting. [p. 42]

Kerr et al. (1978) in *Oral Diagnosis* wrote: "Few will deny that there is an association between nailbiting and tension. When a child or adult feels tense, it is common to see him bite the nails" (p. 51). Although Mitchell (1973) acknowledged the nailbiting-tension connection, he reported that nailbiting is "so common in middle childhood that too much significance should not be attached to . . . [it] at this age" (p. 389).

As reflected in the preceding capsular summary of statements by various writers on the anxiety-nailbiting issue, nailbiting has long been viewed as a behavior that indicates anxiety. Another traditional assumption has been that psychopaths and sociopaths have low anxiety levels. It follows that a low incidence of nailbiting should be found among psychopaths and sociopaths. Walker and Ziskind (1977) observed during several investigations, however, that "the incidence of nailbiting is higher in sociopaths than in either normal controls or patients in other psychiatric categories" (p. 64). In further investigating their observations and the relationship between nailbiting and anxiety, Walker and Ziskind tested 62 outpatient sociopaths and 62 nonsociopathic control subjects. Both groups were matched in terms of age, sex, and intelligence. The Cornell Medical Index Health Questionnaire was administered to the subjects and their answers to the question "Do you bite your nails badly?" were tabulated in order to identify the nailbiters in each group. One shortcoming of this question, as recognized by Walker and Ziskind, was that it did not differentiate nailbiters on the basis of "the degree and duration of the symptom, [or] its intensity" (p. 65), nor did it provide an understanding of factors that affect an individual's nailbiting. Nonetheless, the difference in nailbiting incidence between the two groups, as determined by this question, was significant at the .01 level, with the incidence being twice as high in the sociopathic group (48%) as in the control group (24%). These unexpected findings called into question the traditionally assumed relationship between nailbiting and anxiety.

INTEGRATION HYPOTHESIS

Proponents of the integration hypothesis of nailbiting contend that nailbiting is a symptom that emerges as a result of tension produced by two or more conflicting motivations. An example of such a conflict might be that which arises in a child who feels hostile toward a parent but does not want to reveal his aggression because of his dependency on the parent. He also feels the need to punish himself for his aggressive thoughts. When these two needs, i.e., (1) to aggress against the parent and (2) to deny aggression and punish himself, are expressed at the same time, they can be integrated into the act of nailbiting. The nailbiting enables the individual to express aggression and at the same time to punish himself for his aggressive thoughts.

Writing within a psychoanalytical framework, Manhold (1972) viewed nailbiting as a coping mechanism for hostility. Nailbiting was considered a substitute for and an indirect expression of aggression due to frustration. In this respect, Manhold (1972) stated:

> If an individual's drives, either fundamental or quasi-fundamental, are blocked, frustration occurs. With frustration, rage ensues. Psychoanalytic theory states that the oral cavity, either directly or symbolically, is related to all of the so-called human passions. It is of utmost importance that the individual either satisfy his desires or rid himself of frustration and hostilities. In infancy and childhood, oral drives or desires are given a direct outlet. If a child feels rage he does not hesitate to bite someone or something. Later, in adolescence or adulthood the individual's

> instinctual reactions are suppressed through education to the mores of society, and satisfaction is gained through the use of more appropriate bodily parts or through use of substitute mechanisms. Thus, if a condition of emotional or mental stress should develop in an adolescent or adult and he has been properly indoctrinated into the teachings of his society, he cannot bite or tear at the thing that is causing his frustration. He must find a substitute satisfaction. He may turn to nail-biting, pencil-biting, or other biting or chewing procedures. If this substitute biting is not adequate or if the desire is too strong to be sublimated through this substitution, he will, nevertheless, continue to employ the biting mechanism as a means of gratification for his desire—but he will employ it through more unconscious mechanisms. [p. 174]

Hassin (cited in Viets, 1931) stated:

> Nail-biting is an automatic, unconscious, frequently an impulsive act, a morbid inclination to mutilate the fingers by constantly chewing the nails. It may be combined with . . . other states indicating an abnormal nervous or mental character of the victim. [p. 128]

Bowley (1966) also contended that childhood nailbiting was a coping mechanism for handling aggressive feelings. Bowley wrote that nailbiting shows "a tendency to turn the aggression on to the self, a form of punishment or self-mutilation" (p. 72).

Reports obtained by Hill (1946) from the 100 nailbiters among 223 naval and marine male enlisted personnel who were returned to the U.S. from the Pacific battle area because of nervous conditions revealed that:

> Of the entire group of nail biters, 73% had an unduly irritable disposition. They described their tempers as "quick, violent, high, hot." They said they "get mad real quick," "get mad all at once," "fly off the handle easy," and "flare up and blow up." Among those with unusually irritable natures, only 30% had any civil or naval legal offenses. [p. 185]

Coleman and Seret (1950) studied the role of hostility in fingernail biting behavior. Two groups of undergraduate students participated in the study, with the experimental group consisting of present nailbiters and the control group consisting of individuals who had never bitten their nails. The two groups were matched on age, sex, grade-point average, parents' financial status, and home conditions. The results of the Rosensweig Picture Frustration study revealed a significant difference at the 1% level on extrapunitive, intropunitive, and impunitive factors. As Coleman and Seret (1950) reported:

> Nailbiters had a significantly higher score on impunitiveness than their non-nailbiting controls. That is, nailbiters may be more prone to evade hostility by glossing over the situation and to avoid blame both of themselves and others. [p. 240]

Nailbiters also had a significantly higher score than nonnailbiters on the intropunitive factor. That is, "when hostility is aroused by frustration, nailbiters seem relatively more prone to turn their hostility inward upon themselves" (p. 240). Nonnailbiters showed a greater tendency to "blame external sources for their frustration and to discharge their hostility on to the environment" (p. 240), as indicated by their significantly higher score on extrapunitiveness (Coleman and Seret, 1950).

Upon comparing the experimental and control groups on the basis of their responses to interview questions, Coleman and Seret found that: (a) nailbiters more often felt that they were withholding anger and resentment, even though they realized that it should be released; and (b) there were no differences between nailbiters and nonnailbiters in the type of situation that aroused their hostility. Coleman and Seret (1950) further commented that:

> The finding that nailbiters more often felt they were holding anger or resentment within themselves, while at the same time evidencing no greater amount of hostility in their daydreams and idle thoughts, would tend to support the view of nailbiting as a method of discharging hostility. [p. 243]

By way of interpretation and inference, Coleman and Seret argued that it is possible that nailbiting symbolically represents "(a) the biting and destruction of one's aggressor, or (b) self-punishment for unethical thoughts, or (c) a combination of the two" (p. 243).

The basic theme of an analysis of nailbiting behavior by Isaacs (1952) favored the anger-hostility interpretation. Isaacs (1952) briefly stated, as follows, her formulation of a hypothesis dealing with the anger-hostility notion of fingernail biting behavior:

> Nails are bitten because they are "bad" nails, because they want to scratch, because they are like biting teeth; and the more jagged and menacing they become by being bitten, the more they have to be bitten—to punish them and prevent them from scratching and biting other people. [p. 436]

The basic premise of this interpretation appears to be that directing hostility towards the jagged fingernails is a self-controlling response that enables the nailbiter to handle his aggressive impulses.

Although Coleman and Seret described several ways in which nail-biters cope with hostility, it was Solomon (1955) who attempted to explain *why* nailbiting helps an individual to cope and adapt under circumstances associated with hostility. Solomon's article, "Nail Biting and the Integrative Process," is perhaps unique since most other studies do no more than note that nailbiting frequently accompanies nervousness and tension. Solomon's primary hypothesis was based on the assumption that emotional tension or anxiety results when the organism is beset by two or more conflicting motivations. When these conflicting motivations "are expressed at the same time they can be integrated in the single compulsive act of nail biting" (Solomon, 1955, p. 394). Solomon further elaborated on his hypothesis:

> The integrative aspect of the symptom [nailbiting] consists of the release of oral-sadistic impulses by *biting at the claws.* Thus the release of hostile aggression is accomplished in the biting at the nails which wish to claw. At the same time the external object is spared by engaging the claws. In this way both the need to bite and the need to inhibit the infliction of damage to the external object are satisfied. Furthermore, a guilt-expiating device is afforded the organism by the infliction of pain upon the self. [p. 393]

In accounting for the reason that nailbiting is a frequently emitted response in reducing tension, Solomon isolated the fact that nailbiting is a motor response: "Some form of motor action [such as nailbiting] is a more likely method of release of tension than the more highly conceptualized defences that occur later" (p. 393). Although many forms of motor actions are available to an individual, Solomon suggested that the development of the nailbiting symptom—rather than some other motor response—is favored by the establishment of the hand-mouth relationship early in infancy. Since the infant reaches for objects and puts them to/in his mouth, Solomon contended that the motor responses involved in nailbiting behavior have been present in the behavioral repertoire of most individuals since infancy, except for the final element in the motor sequence, i.e., the act of biting or tearing the nail.

Hand-mouth contact has been observed even prior to infancy in the form of thumb-sucking. Lennart Wilson, a Swedish photographer, clearly illustrates an 18-week-old fetus sucking its thumb in one of his photographs of the human embryo and fetus in an article entitled "Drama of Life Before Birth" in the April 30, 1965, issue of *Life*. This developmental milestone appears to provide additional support to Solomon's discussion of an early hand-mouth relationship.

An impromptu statement by an adolescent nailbiter in a study by Billig (1941) reflected a similar view concerning the etiology of nailbiting. In response to the experimenter's request to try to recall any experience he may have had that was pertinent to nailbiting, the boy replied: "I think the cause of finger nail-biting is from putting your fingers in your mouth when you were a baby. Another cause is as a result of teething" (p. 183).

A recurring theme in Solomon's (1955) discussion is that "nailbiting, which had been a source of comfort, becomes a method in itself for . . . relief . . . in the face of conflictual or tension-provoking situations" (p. 395). The explanation posited by Shahovitch for the occurrence of nailbiting seems to align with Solomon's discussion of the early establishment of certain motor responses. Concerning the mechanism involved in this process, Shahovitch (1945) explained:

> A pattern has been established in . . . [the child's] nervous system which is permanent and may reappear at any time in his life after prolonged or undue strain. The pathway of this habit pattern has been made over his nervous system and can never be entirely obliterated. [p. 303]

According to Shahovitch, the child reacts to anxiety and fear by bringing his hands to his face, a primitive, innate gesture. An analogy was drawn between a beast in terror who will gnaw when he cannot fight and a child in apprehension who brings his hands to his face and "soon learns to gnaw" (p. 303).

An argument almost identical to Solomon's was cogently outlined by Pierce (1975). Although the examination of the integrative function is limited to the quoted passage which follows, it is the primary hypothesis included in his discussion of the etiology of nailbiting:

> The nail biting is thought to be caused by intense or competitive impulses toward a parent. If such impulses were actualized, the child would destroy his source of dependency gratification. To resolve this conflict, the child bites his nails, thus denying his hostility, injuring himself, and demonstrating his punishment. At the same time, he is able to express aggression but spare the object of his aggression. [Pierce, 1975, pp. 2125-2126]

The two pages devoted to a discussion of nailbiting in the February 2, 1974, issue of *Woman* focused on the integrative function of nailbiting, with specific reference to the views of a psychologist named Louis Schendler. The reader was introduced to a suggested etiology of nailbiting by the following statement: "You might think we do it [bite our nails] because we're nervous. But it's not so much a matter of calming our nerves as fighting the demon in us" ("Why Take It Out On Your Nails?," p. 50). Schendler regarded nailbiting as a sign of aggression (p. 50). He went on to argue that nailbiting helps the individual to control his aggression. The integrative function of nailbiting was described as follows:

> Forced to sit still, we get frustrated. One response to frustration is aggression. But we learn by experience that aggression won't get us what we need–love, recognition, acceptance by others. . . . So we "take it out" on our nails. In doing so, we achieve several goals at once: relieve the tension of muscles held in check that leads to aggression; reinforce our body image by proving to ourselves by physical action that we still exist. By finding an outlet for aggression, we're able to keep it to ourselves, avoid antagonizing others–"stay friends." ["Why Take It Out On Your Nails?", p. 50]

Koch (1935) attempted to study the association between mannerisms and behavior patterns suggestive of conflict, escape, and aggression. Inherent in her rationale was the recognition that mannerisms are often referred to as indices of nervousness, which in turn is often regarded as an emotional state resulting from conflict. For the purpose of her study, Koch (1935) defined aggression in terms of three different types of attack:

1. Vigorous "physical attack" included "pushing, pulling, pulling hair, striking, biting, pinching . . . and snatching another's possessions directly from him" (p. 156).

2. "Verbal attack" consisted of "swearing, criticizing, calling names, passing derogatory remarks, ostracising another from the group, contradicting, threatening, gloating, being insolent, expressing doubt of another's convictions, teasing, bullying, tattling, and asserting ownership to ward off competitors" (p. 156).

3. "Indirect attack"–The primary criterion for responses of indirect attack was "inconveniencing an opponent in ways not involving direct physical or verbal assault" (p. 156). Indirect attack included "protecting a possession by reaching for it or covering it before others had a chance to claim it, pursuing another but not attacking, destroying a possession when its owner was absent, and snatching an object when its possessor had his back turned" (pp. 156, 159).

Data analysis (Koch, 1935) revealed a consistently negative correlation between all categories of attack and the frequency of occurrence of digital mannerisms (finger play) for both boys and girls. An examination of the relationship between attack and oral mannerisms such as "sucking, biting, or chewing on things not intended for consumption" (Koch, 1935, p. 140) also generally revealed a low negative correlation for both males and females, with the exception of a positive correlation between indirect attack and oral mannerisms for girls. Pouting and sulking, "attack which is not overt," correlated positively and "probably to a significant degree with a disposition to indulge in finger play" (Koch, 1935, p. 160) and to oral mannerisms for both boys and girls. As postulated by Koch, pouting and sulking were indicative of internal conflict. Interestingly, finger play revealed a larger negative coefficient with the measures of aggressive or conflict behavior than did the other mannerisms. In other words, aggressive behaviors were associated with absence of or minimal finger play (Koch, 1935).

The relationship between compliant behavior and digital and oral mannerisms was also investigated by Koch. She felt that information relating to these traits would shed some light on the understanding of the place of aggression in the behavior of children. Compliant behavior was measured in terms of the child's "accession to requests made of him" (p. 161). Low negative correlations were found between compliant behavior and finger play for boys and girls. A plausible explanation for this finding as put forth by Koch was that the compliant child may be so busy fulfilling requests that he has little time for finger play. Perhaps even more pertinent is the possible direct involvement of the hands in the task, which would preclude finger play. A low positive correlation was indicated between compliance and oral mannerisms.

Table 19 summarizes a portion of the data from Koch, 1935, pertaining to the relationships between digital and oral mannerisms and behavior patterns suggestive of conflict, escape, attack, aggression, and compliance.

CONSISTENCY THEORY OF NAILBITING

The basic premise of Lecky's self-consistency theory was summarized by F. C. Thorne in the foreword to the second edition (1961) of Lecky's *Self-Consistency: A Theory of Personality*:

Table 19 Correlations Between Digital and Oral Mannerisms and Measures of Social Behavior

Measure of social behavior	*Digital (boys)*	*Digital (girls)*	*Oral*
Physical attack	-.541	-.260	-.091
Verbal attack	-.021	-.269	-.210
Indirect attack (boys)	-.347	–	-.081
Indirect attack (girls)	–	-.295	+.140
Pouting or sulking	+.352	+.299	+.111
Complying with requests	-.299	-.060	+.005
Playing alone	-.175	-.248	-.008
Watching others	+.306	+.531	-.084

Adapted from "An Analysis of Certain Forms of So-called 'Nervous Habits' in Young Children," by H. L. Koch, *Journal of Genetic Psychology*, 1935, *46*, 139-170. Copyright by the Journal Press and reprinted with permission.

> The essence . . . [of an individual's] organization of ideas and attitudes is . . . [his] self-consistency. A person can only go in one direction at a time, or believe one thing at a time. Inconsistency or ambivalence results in conflict or paralysis of action. Behavior expresses the effort to be consistent and unified in organization and action. Ideas which are consistent with past experience tend to be assimilated; those which are inconsistent tend to be rejected. If an inconsistent attitude presents itself with sufficient urgency, it may force re-organization of preexisting attitudes in order to eliminate inconsistency and regain unity. [Lecky, p. 3]

Lecky did not apply his theory specifically to nailbiting. He asserted, however, that the trend of decreased thumb-sucking with increasing chronological age aligned with the view expressed in his model. He wrote that:

> Every year millions of children who have industriously sucked their thumbs since birth, and who have successfully resisted every effort to change their behavior, quit the practice spontaneously when they are five or six years old. The reason is that they are beginning at this age to think of themselves as big boys or girls, and they recognize that thumb-sucking is inconsistent with the effort to maintain this new idea. The changed conception of who they are, and the necessity of making good in the new role they have accepted, furnishes them with a new standard to which their behavior must now conform. If a child continues to think of himself as a baby, due perhaps to prolonged illness or overprotection by the parents, the necessary standard is lacking and the thumb-sucking will continue. Parents often invoke the "big boy" standard deliberately in the effort to change the child's behavior in many other situations. [Lecky, pp. 249-250]

Writing in the *Proceedings of the Pennsylvania Academy of Science*, Billig (1946) proposed what might be called a consistency theory of nailbiting. His proposal relied heavily on Lecky's self-consistency theory, which states that "maintaining self-consistency in an unstable environment is of primary importance to an individual" (Billig, 1946, p. 39). In Lecky's words:

> The center or nucleus of the mind is the individual's idea or conception of himself. If a new idea seems to be consistent with the ideas already present in the system, and particularly with the individual's conception of himself, it is accepted and assimilated easily. If it seems to be inconsistent, however, it meets with resistance and is likely to be rejected. This resistance is a natural phenomenon; it is essential for the maintenance of individuality. [Lecky, p. 246]

In extending Lecky's theory to nailbiting, Billig (1946) contended that a habit such as nailbiting will persist only if it is "consistent with the individual's idea of himself" (p. 39). For some individuals, nailbiting may be regarded as being consistent with their self-image in that it is viewed as a helpful coping mannerism that may have "maximum subjective effect by inconspicuous, socially inoffensive means" (Bovet, cited in Billig, 1946, p. 39). Billig (1946) further maintained that during adolescence, social pressures may result in rejection of the nailbiting habit by many individuals. A similar view is embodied in the statement by Bakwin and Bakwin (1968) in their discussion of nailbiting. They noted that "during adolescence the majority of nailbiters, probably influenced by social disapproval, give up the habit" (p. 462). According to Billig (1946), other mannerisms such as smoking and gum-chewing, which have more acceptance by the adult population, are likely to be adopted at this point.

Billig (1946) hypothesized that the proportion of individuals indicating that they were former nailbiters should be consistent or approximately the same over a number of years with different groups of adolescents in the same age group, in the same school situation, and from the same parent population. His hypothesis was supported by the finding that the percentage of nailbiters for each of the 6 years studied appeared to be stable. For those individuals classified as former nailbiters, there was a slight fluctuation, but it was not statistically significant. The number and percentages of nailbiters and former nailbiters are summarized in Table 20, which has been adapted from a detailed presentation of the data by Billig, 1946. Billig interpreted his findings to mean that the former nailbiters "found nailbiting to be inconsistent with their idea of themsel[ves] and have assumed an equivalent mannerism more consistent with their present

Table 20 Distribution of Nailbiters and Former Nailbiters According to Years

Year	*Total N*	*Present nailbiters N*	*Present nailbiters Percent*	*Former nailbiters N*	*Former nailbiters Percent*
1940	190	53	27.9	71	37.4
1941	150	44	29.3	57	38.0
1942	180	50	27.8	67	37.2
1943	150	41	27.3	55	36.7
1944	220	62	28.2	92	41.8
1945	170	46	27.1	68	40.0
Total	1060	296	27.9	410	38.7

Adapted from "The Consistency of Finger-nail Biting," by A. L. Billig, *Proceedings of the Pennsylvania Academy of Science*, 1946, *20*, 39-43. Copyright by the Pennsylvania Academy of Science and reprinted with permission.

idea" (p. 42). It is difficult, however, to see how his data supported this interpretation. First, each subject was simply asked to write his name in one of three columns, thus indicating whether he was a current nailbiter, former nailbiter, or nonnailbiter. Had the investigator asked those persons who said they were former nailbiters to indicate *why* they stopped, additional support may have been given to his hypothesis. Second, there is no indication in Billig's 1946 study that the former nailbiters were questioned to determine whether they adopted another mannerism to replace the nailbiting habit and whether they considered any newly acquired mannerism to be more consistent with their self-image.

Coleman and McCalley (1948b) interpreted "inconsistency" quite differently and therefore questioned Billig's data on different grounds. They commented:

> Billig noted that there was considerable consistency of incidence [of nailbiting among 14- to 16-year-olds over a period of 6 years], which he attributed to the consistency of the individuals within the samples themselves. This is puzzling in view of the

> fact that the samples never used the identical subjects more than once, and hence individual consistency would appear to be a rather meaningless concept. [Coleman and McCalley, 1948b, p. 431]

Massler and Malone (1950) also noted that it is likely that many individuals give up severe nailbiting after the age of 15 and then assume what Billig (1946, p. 42) termed an "equivalent mannerism:"

> Nailbiting originates as a transfer from thumb-sucking some time between 4 and 6 years of age when social (parental) censure demands that sucking habits be discontinued. In turn, nailbiting must be discontinued when society again demands it. Most children successfully resist parental demands to stop nailbiting, but sometime after the age of 15 years the censure of friends makes it expedient for the average gregarious child to substitute some other "habit." [Massler and Malone, p. 525]

To illustrate the substitution of an innocuous habit for the nailbiting mannerism. Massler and Malone asserted that "gumchewing offers a socially acceptable method of oral gratification. In fact, it is a good method of 'transferring' habitual nailbiting. In the adult, smoking is a common nailbiting substitute" (p. 525).

Many of the former nailbiters and nonnailbiters in a study by Coleman and McCalley (1948a) reported that they had developed habits such as "pencil chewing, cigarette smoking, finger tapping, head scratching, doodling, and 'popping' the knuckles of the hands" (p. 520). The subjects regarded these habits as substitutes for nailbiting that "gave them some sort of relief from tension" (p. 520).

Sim and Finn (1973) viewed nailbiting as a harmless habit that "develops after the sucking age" (p. 380). They contended that nailbiting may be a substitute for finger-sucking and also that at a later age chewing gum, pencils, or erasers, or smoking, etc., may become "substitutes for the fingers, for every age has its own pacifiers" (p. 380). An earlier writer (Peck, 1953) proposed that school-age children substitute nailbiting for finger-sucking because the habit of finger-sucking is one "in which they are now ashamed to indulge" (p. 360). Although this orientation appears to overlap with the preceding formulation of a consistency theory of nailbiting, a data base is not stated.

COPING AND EXPRESSIVE FUNCTIONS OF NAILBITING

Allport suggested that the concept of functional autonomy may have a place in a theory of fingernail biting behavior. Allport offered a theoretical distinction for determining whether or not functional autonomy was exhibited in nailbiting by particular individuals:

> If under psychoanalysis the patient relives the past . . . and learns what repressed incidents have been troublesome, and *if this backward training effects a cure* (because the patient sees that the troublesome element has no place in his current motivational system), then the neurosis was *not* functionally autonomous. If, on the other hand, a "character neurosis" is so firmly structured that it now constitutes the life-pattern, and if nothing can dislodge it, then we have no choice but to admit that it is an acquired, functionally autonomous, motivational system. [Allport, 1961, pp. 240-241]

This distinction appears to indicate that in therapy it should be determined whether or not the patient's symptom is functionally autonomous; i.e., whether treatment should focus on the underlying cause (not functionally autonomous) or on a re-education process involving eradication of the problem as it is manifested in observable behavior (functionally autonomous). As Allport stated: "It would seem wise for the therapist to determine whether the patient's symptoms are to be relieved by 'going to the root of the problem' or whether the most that can be hoped for is to reconcile the patient to his own developed style of life" (p. 241). This guideline seems to be puzzling since it implies that treatment, whether in the form of psychoanalysis or symptomatic therapy, must first be applied in order to ascertain the nature of the problem behavior and hence appropriate treatment.

Allport's principle of functional autonomy as applied to nailbiting appears to be partly substantiated by the findings of Pennington and Mearin (1944), at least "at the descriptive level" (p. 631). Many adult male subjects of military age reported that: (a) their habit was acquired in childhood; (b) there were older members in their family who were nailbiters; and (c) they were unaware of their nailbiting acts. Some men were astonished when they observed their own nails. Pennington and Mearin proposed that nailbiting, although a learned act, gradually acquires "its own motivating force" (p. 631). When the childhood need to bite dissipates, the nailbiting continues "without undue external stimulation and without fulfilling any apparent need" (p. 631). The habit "is then said to be functionally autonomous . . . since it has its own drive" and is illustrative of the " 'strangle hold' . . . that an early response pattern can acquire in the absence of the original stimuli" (Pennington and Mearin, 1944, p. 631). Holt and McIntosh (1940) also acknowledged that nailbiting may outlive the behavior disorder with which it was originally associated: "Nailbiting responds slowly; in a period of readjustment other symptoms may disappear long before the nailbiting" (p. 940).

Nailbiters commonly express the fear that their nailbiting may be symptomatic of a personality disorder (Azrin and Nunn, 1977). The view of Azrin and Nunn is that the factors that contribute to the acquisition of a nervous habit, such as imitating others or lack of awareness of the movement, are normal. They also viewed as being normal the anxiety and sensitivity that may result from the nailbiting habit. As they stated:

> Once the habit is gone, most clients report that they feel less anxiety and are more relaxed. You should not feel, therefore, that your nervous habit is a sign of neurosis, but rather that it is probably causing some of the feelings of neurosis. That is, the habit is probably causing the nervousness at least as much as nervousness is causing the habit. [Azrin and Nunn, pp. 37-38]

Pennington and Mearin (1944) stated that two interpretations have been formulated about nailbiting behavior. One of these assumes that nailbiting is suggestive of "unhealthy mental attitudes and of behavior disorders, and is consequently regarded symptomatically" (p. 629). The other, to which Pennington and Mearin adhered, considers nailbiting as an expressive form of body movement that is not symptomatic of an underlying behavior disorder in essentially normal individuals. They contended that nailbiting is often and perhaps inaccurately used as "evidence of whatever its user means by 'nervousness' " (p. 628).

Pennington and Mearin suggested that the manner in which the nailbiter reacts to his own hands and to questions concerning his nailbiting behavior may help the clinician to formulate a tentative hypothesis as to whether the nailbiting is symptomatic or not symptomatic of underlying psychopathology. The likelihood of the presence of other problems is not great if the individual is accepting of his nailbiting behavior. Denial of the habit or an unwillingness to stop nailbiting should be regarded as a clue to other behavioral problems.

If nailbiting is to be regarded as either an expressive type of behavior or a form of coping behavior, it seems relevant to examine the assumptions of each behavior type as well as the distinctions between them. A recognition of these characteristics would help in formulating certain hypotheses concerning the degree of expressive or coping behavior manifested by an individual's nailbiting mannerism. The guidelines would be even more helpful if, in addition, they assisted the clinician in deciding on the general approach or mode of treatment.

Maslow (1949) made several distinctions between expressive and coping behavior. These were also included in Allport's discussion in his 1961 revision of *Pattern and Growth in Personality*. As outlined by Maslow (1949):

1. Coping is by definition purposive and motivated; expression is most often unmotivated.
2. Coping is more determined by environmental and cultural variables; expression is largely determined by the state of the organism. A corollary is the much higher correlation of expression with deep-lying character structure.
3. Coping is most often learned ["formally elicited" (Allport, 1961)]; expression most often unlearned ["spontaneously emitted" (Allport, 1961)].
4. Coping is more easily controlled (repressed, suppressed, inhibited, acculturated); expression is often uncontrolled and even uncontrollable.
5. Coping is usually designed to cause changes in the environment and often does; expression is not "designed" to do anything. If it causes environmental changes, it does so unwittingly.
6. Coping is characteristically means-behavior, the end being need-gratification or threat-reduction. Expression is often an end-in-itself.
7. Typically, the coping component is conscious (although it

may become unconscious); expression is more often not conscious. [pp. 261-262]

In his book, *Motivation and Personality*, Maslow (1970) presented basically the same distinctions, but included one more:

8. Coping is effortful; expression is effortless in most instances. Artistic expression is of course a special and in-between case, because one *learns* to be spontaneous and expressive (if one is successful). One can *try* to relax. [p. 132]

Nailbiting was described by Smith (1957) in the light of the theoretical formulation of the expressive component of behavior as outlined by Maslow (1949). Smith recognized that nailbiting among college students may initially have been a form of coping behavior; that is, a means of reducing tension. In the majority of college student nailbiters, Smith proposed that nailbiting is a form of expressive rather than coping behavior; that is, the "habit" has persisted even after the underlying cause has ceased to be operative (p. 219). At the same time, he acknowledged that in some instances the underlying cause persists and hence accounts for the continuation of the nailbiting. Smith's hypothesis that nailbiting is a form of expressive behavior was based on the results of a study by Dunlap (1932/1972). Dunlap found that within a group of college students who were all severe nailbiters, every student broke the biting habit within three weeks as a result of 20 minutes per day of symptomatic treatment in the form of negative practice. Smith interpreted this finding to mean that nailbiting is an expressive type of behavior among many college students. He reasoned that if it were a form of coping behavior, symptomatic treatment would not effectively end the nailbiting. Smith recognized, however, that his interpretation would be valid only if the number of relapses among Dunlap's subjects were minimal. Unfortunately, Dunlap did not report on the number of subjects who returned to nailbiting after completing treatment.

Smith also attempted to examine the effectiveness of symptomatically treating nailbiting among college students. Smith's study supported the hypothesis that nailbiting among college students is often an expressive habit that can be symptomatically treated, especially in individuals between the ages of 19 and 21. The study bridges the gap between armchair theorizing about the expressive nature of nailbiting and empirical testing of the effectiveness of symptomatic treatment of nailbiting.

Maberly (1943) stated that psychological problems in childhood are "frequent in occurrence, numerous in type, and variable in character" (p. 362), adding that a child may make no complaints about a particular behavior (e.g., nailbiting), but because parents or teachers complain, it is often considered a behavioral problem. Concerning diagnosis and treatment, Maberly contended that it should first be ascertained whether the problem is mainly psychological or physical in nature as well as in origin; that is, whether the problem is mainly a "constitutional defect . . . an acquired defect . . . [or] a simple environmental maladjustment" (p. 362). Maberly interpreted his phrase "psychological in origin" to mean "emotional stress arising from inner conflict . . . or from some alteration in the environment to which the child has been unable to adapt" (p. 362). A second general guideline suggested by Maberly in determining the nature and origin of the problem is "the occasion on which the symptom first appeared, and the circumstances in which subsequent attacks developed. Equally should enquiries elicit any purpose served, what satisfaction might be gained" (p. 363).

If an underlying disturbance is responsible for the behavior and if it is correctly diagnosed and treated, "results can be immediate and dramatic," Maberly noted (p. 363). Symptomatic treatment in this instance, according to Maberly, is rarely of value. In specifically relating this statement to nailbiting, Maberly suggested that nailbiting is often indicative of insecurity and frustration in the child and if the nailbiting is to be cured, "both factors [insecurity and frustration] must be recognized and dealt with so far as possible" (p. 365). Another point in Maberly's discussion of the treatment of nailbiting was that the age of onset may be helpful in identifying the underlying emotional conflict. Although Maberly's suggestions concerning the diagnosis and treatment of underlying disturbances that may be responsible for the nailbiting were well intentioned, their descriptive impreciseness renders them too general to be useful as prescriptive diagnostic and remedial strategies.

With regard to the coping-expressive behavior issue, Sherbon (1941) wrote: "If the habit has a neurotic basis and becomes intractable, the nervous child's real trouble is much more serious than the overt act of biting the nails, which is only a minor symptom of deeper difficulty–usually only one of numerous symptoms" (p. 577). If nailbiting is a symptom of deeper difficulty, it would appear that symptomatic treatment procedures would be inappropriate for this habit.

Two of Pringle's (1974) five criteria of behavioral maladjustment in children related to the "intensity and the persistence of a particular symptom" (p. 72). In illustrating the significance of the intensity of a symptom, specific reference was made to nailbiting: "Research has shown that the great majority of children bite their nails at some time or other. However, few do it to the extent of drawing blood. Such a degree of intensity indicates emotional disturbance rather than just a bad habit" (Pringle, 1974, p. 72). Her criteria of intensity and persistence seem to align with the philosophies of Anthony (1970) and Azrin and Nunn (1977), who considered the intensity, frequency, and persistence of nailbiting to be pertinent to an examination of the behavior.

In attempting to empirically support the contention that nailbiting is not symptomatic of a deeper behavior disorder, Pennington and Mearin (1944) examined the frequency and significance of nailbiting among 2,297 naval recruits. Their study was conducted by observing the extended hands of recruits at the outset of a 5-minute neuropsychiatric and psychological examination. The data were obtained for each subject by closely inspecting "the nail of each finger on the two hands" (p. 629). In addition, it was also recorded whether each examinee passed the brief neurological, psychiatric, and psychological tests or whether further examination was required. No attempt was made to group nailbiters according to the number of fingernails bitten or the severity of the nailbiting. An individual was designated as a nailbiter as long as there was evidence of biting "the nail of a single finger" (Pennington and Mearin, p. 629).

In discussing their results, Pennington and Mearin indicated that "only 27 per cent of the nail-biters were required to undergo more detailed neuropsychiatric and psychological examinations" (p. 629). The data summary in Table 21 reports only 9.75% of the nailbiters as being required to undergo further psychiatric examination; that is, 51 out of the 533 nailbiters. The 27% appears to refer to the percentage of nailbiters among the total number of recruits held over for

Table 21 Frequency of Nailbiting Among 2,297 Naval Recruits

Nailbiters	*"Hold-over" total*	*Nailbiters among those "held over"*
Number 533	192	51
Percent 23.20	8.36	26.56 percent (192 cases) 9.75 percent (533 cases) 2.20 percent (2,297 cases)

From "The Frequency and Significance of a Movement Mannerism for the Military Psychiatrist," by L. A. Pennington and R. J. Mearin, *American Journal of Psychiatry*, 1944, *100*, 628-632. Copyright by the American Psychiatric Association and reprinted with permission.

further psychiatric assessment; that is, of the total number of 192 recruits who were held over, 51 were nailbiters. The fact that the percentage of nailbiters requiring further examination is actually only 9.75% even further supports the statement by Pennington and Mearin that "numerous recruits, addicted in degree to nail-biting, revealed no other neurological, psychiatric or psychological symptoms sufficient, in terms of present standards of military selection, to disqualify them" (p. 629). Actually, this group represented about 90% of the 533 nailbiters, which may be interpreted as supporting Pennington and Mearin's hypothesis that nailbiting is an expressive form of body movement, not symptomatic of underlying behavior disorders. Table 21 summarizes the frequency of nailbiting among the recruits in their study.

Pennington and Mearin concluded that nailbiting is not always indicative of the existence of a "psychoneurotic or other abnormal condition" but may merely be a reflection of the fact that "habits often outlast their inciting conditions" (p. 631). Nailbiting may have at one time fulfilled a need, but it gradually acquires "its own motivating force" (p. 631) and hence is usually considered to be functionally autonomous, they noted.

Peck (1953) noted that although the cause of a habit such as nailbiting may be eliminated, this "does not always automatically remove the habit" (p. 361). This statement seems to reflect the opinion of Pennington and Mearin. Bakwin (1971) was another dissenting voice against the widespread view that nailbiting is a manifestation of psychopathology. One argument that he advanced against this popular proposition was the fact that "relinquishing the habit during adolescence is not known to be accompanied by the substitution of other neurotic manifestations" (Bakwin, 1971, p. 307).

ENVIRONMENTAL RESTRICTION MODEL

Bethell (1958) has suggested that nailbiting and other tension habits in children could be related to restriction in the child's environment. The living conditions of the family, the personalities of the child's parents, and discord in the parent's marital relationship were considered by Bethell to be the main contributors to this environmental restriction. With regard to the personalities of the child's parents, Bethell identified the following traits as being restrictive factors: "anxiety, irritability, depression, rigidity and an overtly restrictive or over-protective attitude" (pp. 264-265). In identifying the family conditions that were considered sources of restriction in the child's environment, Bethell specified the following: "flat [apartment] dwelling, overcrowding, the presence of restricting neighbours and the absence of a garden" (p. 265). The size of the child's family was not included as one of these factors, since Bethell considered this condition to be indirectly related to overcrowding.

In investigating the relationship between nailbiting and restriction in the environment, Bethell obtained the case histories of 100 children ranging in age from 3 to 15 years who attended the Children's Department of the Maudsley Hospital, London, England. In outlining the specific experimental procedure, Bethell stated:

> Firstly, case histories were obtained of fifty children in whom one or more of the habits of nail biting, nose picking, and head banging had been recorded as an established practice. From these case histories the information about the presence of restrictive factors was obtained. Secondly, in order to be able to evaluate by statistical methods any apparently high incidence of restrictive elements that might be found in the environment of the selected children who showed the tension habits, another fifty case histories of problem children in whom these habits had not been observed, were obtained. [p. 265]

Bethell reported that the number of times the 12 restrictive items occurred in the experimental (tension) group was approximately four times their occurrence in the control group. The difference between the mean number of items for the experimental group (4.42) and the control group (1.64) was significant beyond the .1% level. The findings are summarized in Table 22.

In evaluating the findings, Bethell cautioned:

> The high incidence of restrictive factors found, however, does not mean that these are directly causal, because they might be due to differences in other, uncontrolled variables. For example, children in the tension group might have been ones who had been physically ill at an early age, and this on the one hand might have caused tension habits and on the other hand might have turned their mothers into restrictive ones. [p. 267]

Table 22 Frequency of Occurrence of Twelve Restrictive Items in Home Environment of Nailbiters

Item	*Tension group*	*Control group*
Father		
1. Anxious	5	2
2. Depressed, irritable	24	9
3. Rigid	4	0
4. Restrictive	9	2
Mother		
5. Depressed, irritable	25	7
6. Rigid	2	2
7. Over-protective and restrictive	28	9
8. Disturbed marital relationship	19	7
Accommodation		
9. Flat [Apartment]	40	19
10. Overcrowded	19	8
11. Neighbors restrictive	15	2
12. No garden	31	2
Totals	221	82

From "Restriction and Habits in Children," by M. F. Bethell, *Zeitschrift Kinderpsychiatry*, 1958, *25*, 264-269. Copyright by Verlag Schwabe and Company and reprinted with permission.

Schendler (cited in "Why Take It Out On Your Nails?," 1974) argued that restriction of motor behavior, such as prolonged sitting in school, interferes with a child's body image. He specifically offered the view that:

> This [sitting still] affects the functioning of our "body image" —a kind of model in our minds of our shape, position, shape in space. We *know* we exist when we're moving around—we can *feel* we do. But when we're forced to sit still we have to reassure ourselves—play with our hair, scratch or rub our skin, bite our nails—provoke sensations that keep us aware of our body. [p. 50]

AZRIN AND NUNN'S EXPLANATION FOR FINGERNAIL BITING AND ITS PERSISTENCE

In identifying the factors that contribute to the acquisition of nervous habits, Azrin and Nunn (1977) claimed that habits such as thumbsucking and nailbiting had their beginnings in normal behavior. A mannerism becomes a problem only when it occurs at a high frequency or persists beyond the period of normalcy. Azrin and Nunn (1977) stated:

> Virtually all children suck either on a bottle or on their mother's breast during infancy, and the thumb-sucking habit is simply a continuation of a nearly universal and normal activity. Nail biting often starts because of irregularities of the nail or cuticle. . . . Many people . . . began to imitate a family member who had the habit. All of these causes or antecedents are entirely normal. The great persistence or high frequency of the mannerism is what makes it a problem. [p. 33]

According to Azrin and Nunn (1973), the factors that contribute to the persistence of nervous habits, including nailbiting, are "response chaining, limited awareness, excessive practice and social tolerance" (p. 619). The following statement sets forth the details of their formulation:

> The present rationale is that a nervous habit originally starts as a normal reaction. The reaction may be to an extreme event such as a physical injury or psychological trauma (see also Yates, 1970), or the symptom may have started as an infrequent, but

> normal, behavior that has increased in frequency and been altered in its form. The behavior becomes classified as a nervous habit when it persists after the original injury or trauma has passed and when it assumes an unusual form and unusually high frequency. Under normal circumstances the nervous habit would be inhibited by personal or social awareness of its peculiarity or by its inherent inconvenience. The movement may, however, have blended into normal movements so gradually as to escape personal and social awareness. Once having achieved this transformation, the movement is performed so often as to become a strongly established habit that further escapes personal awareness because of its automatic nature. . . . This analysis of nervous habits suggests several methods of treatment. The client should learn to be aware of every occurrence of the habit. Each habit movement should be interrupted so that it no longer is part of a chain of normal movements. A physically competing response should be established to interfere with the habit. [p. 620]

Azrin and Nunn's 1977 explanation for the persistence of fingernail biting was similar to their 1973 rationale and was based on several assumptions:

1. Nailbiting is acquired gradually. The individual becomes accustomed to the annoyances of the habit because the progression from "occurring only occasionally" to "occurring frequently" (p. 34) is a gradual one that takes place over a period of months or even years.

2. The nailbiter is often unaware that he is biting his fingernails and hence is unaware of the frequency with which he bites. The emphasis in Azrin and Nunn's (1977) treatment procedures, therefore, was on increasing the individual's awareness of each instance of nailbiting.

3. The absence of social reaction prevents the individual from realizing that others are bothered by his nailbiting. Social reaction may be absent because of a sympathetic attitude on the part of friends and strangers who wish not to embarrass the nailbiter and hence pretend unawareness (p. 36). Consequently, Azrin and Nunn (1977) recommended in one aspect of their treatment program that the nailbiter ask a friend to remind him that his habit is very noticeable.

4. Nailbiting becomes intertwined with other behaviors such as

reading, talking, driving a car, and listening. As a result of these associations, the nailbiting occurs whenever the individual is engaging in one of these activities.

Included in Azrin and Nunn's treatment program were specific guidelines for separating the nailbiting mannerism from its associated behaviors. These are discussed in Chapter 5.

DISCOMFORT THEORY

Bevans identified the cause of children's nailbiting as the discomfort associated with poorly manicured fingernails. According to her "discomfort theory," children's play often results in dirty hands, dry and rough skin around the fingernails, broken nails, and the acquisition of hangnails. It is only natural that the child would want to "nip off these troublesome ends" (Bevans, 1945, p. 58). Care of the nails and cuticles, therefore, seems to be a logical preventive measure for nailbiting. As Bevans remarked: "Illogical as it may seem, one of the most successful preventives, and also cures of the habit once it has started, is actual care of the nails and cuticle" (p. 58).

Nailbiting and other oral habits may play a different role in reducing discomfort. From the point of view of Barnett, an individual may discover by random and accidental movements that putting his finger in his mouth helps to ease the discomfort associated, for example, with teething or gingivitis. Barnett provided a detailed outline of the potential development of some oral habits through such a random and accidental process:

> Some random behaviors do, however, have origins that may be so clinically remote that they may not be identified. For example, an infant might have suffered from discomfort caused by teething as the maxillary incisors were erupting. To relieve the pain, he might have rubbed the gums with his thumb. Having found that this pressure anesthesia was comforting, he might have held his thumb against the sore maxillary gingiva. Soon, he might have begun to regularly suck his thumb because he found it to his liking. In other words, in this particular child's case, the placement of the finger in the mouth is an example of random behavior. Relief of distress from teething could have also been

achieved by chewing on a hard cracker, by being given a general oral analgesic, or by using a topical anesthetic. This child happened to find relief when he put his finger in his mouth. Some children may discover the pleasure of finger sucking when they put their finger in their mouth after it was injured from a cut or a burn. This random behavior could initiate a nocive oral behavior. However, clinically it is often too remote to detect.

The purpose here is to indicate that not every behavior has deep-rooted, imitative physical or emotional causes. Behaviors that were originally random usually respond more rapidly to therapy. [Barnett, 1974, p. 221]

THE ROLE OF IMITATION*

With regard to the etiology of nailbiting, Langford stated: "The [nailbiting] habit tends to occur in many members of the same family, and imitation seems to be a factor in its genesis" (1972, p. 276). Billig found that nailbiters frequently claimed to have learned their habit by observing another indulger. Billig reported that the following conclusions, although tentative, would seem warranted:

> Nail-biting is essentially a learned behavior developing, however, on the basis of predispositions which are not common or constant in all individuals. In our culture this behavior is not formally taught; however, some of the students indicated that they started this form of behavior by choice after having observed someone else indulging in it. If the individual indulging possessed status, as far as the observer was concerned, and the observer possessed suitable (emotional) predispositions, the learning of nail-biting followed. In this way the former individual unintentionally taught this behavior to the latter. [1941, p. 150]

*Observational learning may be a more appropriate term. Observational learning occurs when a child observes a model's behavior but performs no observable responses nor receives direct reinforcing consequences himself. To illustrate modeling effects, learning must be distinguished from performance. The requirement for learning via modeling is the observation of a model. Whether or not a learned response is performed seems to depend on the consequences associated with the observed responses of the model. In addition, the imitation of a model depends on such factors as the status, expertise, and prestige of the model, the number of models observed, and the similarity of the model to the observer.

The responses by secondary school students to the inquiry as to whether there is "anything you can remember of when, and how, you started to bite your nails?" (Billig, 1941, p. 144), suggest that modeling was implicated in developing the nailbiting mannerism. The verbatim transcripts of the students' responses revealed a tendency for the development of nailbiting behavior to be connected with observing another person engaging in the act of nailbiting. Representative answers to the question were:

> I began to bite my nails at the beginning of last year. I saw someone else bite them, so I began to bite them. I was excited.
>
> I learned to bite my nails from my sister and brother.
>
> My girl friend bit her nails, so I did.
>
> I started because when I became nervous I could not resist the temptation. I learned from my brother.
>
> I learned from another girl, I watched her, then I started it too. I bite them every time I get a spanking. . . .
>
> I learned from my playmate, when I started school. I bite them because I am nervous. . . .
>
> I started to bite my nails last year. I saw almost all the girls in our club do it so I did it too. [Billig, 1941, pp. 147-148]

According to Hill (1946), 25% of the 100 nailbiters in his study "had parents or older siblings who were nail biters" (p. 185). Illingworth (1964) made reference to the modeling influence as a possible cause of nailbiting: "In some cases nail-biting may perhaps result from imitation of others" (p. 51). Kanner (1972), in the fourth edition to *Child Psychiatry*, offered his opinion on this matter, based on clinical experience:

> Tension is especially apt to express itself in the form of nail biting if the pattern has been furnished by older members of the family. We often had the experience, when inquiring about the existence of this habit in the patient, that the parent stated: "Yes, he does that, but I have always done that myself." One mother said: "He bites his fingernails constantly. Of course, I do that myself. I don't know whether he takes after me or whether it is caused from his nervousness." [p. 529]

Azrin and Nunn (1977) reported that "many people state that they unconsciously began to imitate a family member who had the habit" (p. 33). Azrin and Nunn viewed occasional nailbiting in such instances as being nonproblematic.

A number of relevant observations were provided by the nurses in the children's ward of the hospital where Billig (1941) carried out his investigation. In this study, each nurse was assigned to observe and report on two nailbiters. Billig (1941) felt that the evidence submitted by the nurses was contaminated by their tendency to state their opinions rather than report the facts. He nonetheless included three of the nurses' reports in his paper. A statement submitted by one nurse stressed the therapeutic effects of drawing attention to her own fingernails, which were once bitten. In the nurse's words: "I showed them my nails as I used to bite my own nails, and it seemed to work in keeping them from biting theirs" (Billig, 1941, p. 169). Analysis of this strategy appeared to reveal two components. First, the encouraging coping component; i.e., "I used to bite my own nails." Second, a positive visual model of the nurse's nonnailbitten fingers. This may be the first indication in the published nailbiting literature of a positive visual model (showing the favorable consequences of *not* biting) being deliberately used in hopes of changing the nailbiter's behavior.

Billig attempted to determine what methods, if any, had been used by nailbiters to curb their own nailbiting behavior. A 15-year-old girl's elaboration of her attempts to stop nailbiting were given: "I just stopped biting my fingernails because I thought of how some girls had nice nails and I always looked at mine to compare and I'd think of what an ugly thing it was to do at my age" (Billig, 1941, p. 175). An excerpt from a 12-year-old girl's case history was also presented: "Left institution a few days after treatment started, but during that time had completely stopped biting her nails. Her nails were well manicured, and clean. Saw someone with nice nails and she decided she wanted her nails to look like theirs" (p. 167). Although the modeling proposition is usually discussed in terms of its role in the onset of nailbiting, these two illustrations extend the modeling concept to a consideration of its possible role in helping individuals to desist nailbiting.

Bakwin offered what may be considered a critique of the modeling-nailbiting issue:

> The habit is markedly familial. In a large percentage of cases a history of nail-biting during childhood by one or both of the parents can be obtained. It has been suggested that the children learn to bite the nails by imitating the parents, but this cannot be the case since parents usually stop the habit before their children are born. [1971, p. 304]

Bakwin has empirically examined the question of a genetic basis for nailbiting behavior. His investigation revealed that "MZ [monozygotic] twins are concordant for the habit about twice as often as DZ [dizygotic] twins" (1971, p. 306). With regard to severe nailbiting, monozygotic twins "were concordant more than four times as often as DZ [dizygotic] twins" (p. 306), an even more striking difference. Bakwin did not limit his studies to nailbiting among twins. Data that he obtained on the parents and siblings of nailbiting twins provided further evidence for a genetic basis for nailbiting. It was found that "the closer the genetic relationship, the greater the likelihood of the relative also being a nail-biter" (Bakwin and Bakwin, 1972, p. 510). In addition, the author of the original study, H. Bakwin (1971), reported that "although parents, with few exceptions, had ceased biting their nails before their children were born, the incidence in the children of parents who had been nail-biters was almost three times as great as when neither parent had been a nail-biter" (p. 307).

ROUGH-EDGE NAILBITING HYPOTHESIS

In discussing the specific causes of nailbiting, Azrin and Nunn (1977) included the issue of the visual-kinesthetic stimulus of the rough fingernail edge. They put it this way: "Nail biting often starts because of irregularities of the nail or cuticle" (p. 33). Sherbon (1941) proposed that in most cases, keeping the nail free of rough edges would eliminate the nailbiting. According to Sherbon, nailbiting "may occur . . . in any child whose nails are not properly cared for" (p. 577). To further emphasize her position on this issue, she added:

> It is highly irritating to have rough, snaggy nails that catch on fabrics. Some persons have such sensitive nail beds that they cannot tolerate the friction and instinctively try to smooth the edges of the nails with the teeth. A visit to a manicurist and pro-

> vision of a suitable personal manicure outfit, with careful watching that the nail edges are kept smooth and closely filed, will practically always lead to the habit's fading. [Sherbon, 1941, p. 577]

Bakwin and Bakwin (1972) recognized that a rough fingernail edge may entice the nailbiter and recommended: "The nail-biter should always carry a nail file, since a rough nail is a well-nigh irresistible invitation to bite" (p. 510).

Guthrie (1938) emphasized the stimulus aspect of nailbiting behavior:

> The cue for the action [nailbiting] may have been the feeling of the rough edge of the nail and the removal of this cue may stop the habit, particularly when the nail is now strongly associated with the visit to the manicur[ist] and a new attitude toward nails. [pp. 149-150]

Billig (1941) questioned Guthrie's position on the rough edge and stated that rarely is the rough nail edge a sufficient condition for nailbiting to occur. For the following reason, he suggested the cautious use of the manicure treatment for nailbiting: "When manicuring is used, it should be given judiciously or it may become incorporated as part of the nailbiting syndrome" (p. 203). Guthrie was not proposing, however, that the rough edge was an adequate stimulus for nailbiting. In his chapter entitled "The Description of Personalities," Guthrie used the example of nailbiting to illustrate that personality traits can be measured to some extent by examining an individual's past. Habits and interests are a part of this past and since "repetitiousness is one of the outstanding features of conduct" (p. 149), habits and interests seem to persist. Guthrie (1938) cited some examples: "The lazy scholar tends to remain a lazy scholar. The nail-biter continues to bite his nails" (p. 149). Although Guthrie stated that "we are generally fairly safe in judging an individual's future by his past" (p. 149), he emphasized that the past is of no value to the psychologist who is trying to rid a person of an annoying habit. As Guthrie stated:

> His past now gives no information because it has no record of his behavior under altered conditions. Only the observation of other persons who have been subjected to some form of inter-

> ference will answer this question. It is in this case that the psychologist's information about the nature of learning and his observation of other persons prove of some use. He may have discovered that nail-biters who have been sent to a manicurist for a number of regular visits give up their bad habit. The cue for the action may have been the feeling of the rough edge of the nail and the removal of this cue may stop the habit, particularly when the nail is now strongly associated with the visit to the manicur[ist] and a new attitude toward nails. The psychologist may not have the intimate and prolonged acquaintance that makes it possible to foretell behavior in detail, but he has a larger equipment of observation and record of many persons in typical situations. If he can recognize and classify types of persons, he has an opportunity to make rules for such types. [pp. 149-150]

Thus it can be seen that Guthrie's example was merely illustrating an "if-and-suppose" situation; i.e., if a psychologist discovered that nail-biters stopped biting after making regular visits to a manicurist, it could be supposed that the condition of the fingernails was a critical factor in the previous continuation of the habit.

If tactile-kinesthetic cues play a role at all in nailbiting, they must await the development of the finger prehension response. According to Bayley (cited in Jersild, Telford, and Sawrey, 1975), fine prehension, the ability to pick up "a small pellet precisely with thumb and forefinger" (p. 155), develops between the eighth and tenth month. Prior to this age, it seems reasonable that the child would experience difficulty in feeling the nail edges with the thumb. In addition, unless the child has developed sufficiently in dentition, he would be unable to bite his fingernails. The child would not have a full complement of deciduous teeth until approximately 24 months of age. The lower limit in chronological age for nailbiting therefore appears to be established by dentition, although it seems possible that the child may become aware of his rough nail edges before his dentition had matured sufficiently to enable biting. It may not be necessary, however, for a child to have acquired all of his teeth before being able to bite his fingernails. An 18-month-old child, for example, was observed by Illingworth (1964, p. 51) to be a nailbiter. Although not specified by Illingworth, this nailbiter may have been a girl, since the usual trend in the maturation of dentition is for girls to acquire teeth earlier than boys (Stott, 1967).

MOTOR LEARNING THEORY

As stated by Solomon (1955), a likely outlet for nervous tension is some kind of motor response. Solomon posited that the response selected by the individual is most likely to be nailbiting because of the establishment of the hand-mouth relationship early in infancy. Researchers such as Perkins and Perkins (1976) and Azrin and Nunn (1977) also placed emphasis on the motoric aspect of their treatment procedures. In fact, the target behavior in many contemporary studies of the treatment of nailbiting is often a selected aspect in the chain of motor responses that comprise the nailbiting act; e.g., raising the hand toward the mouth (Azrin and Nunn, 1977; Daniels, 1974) or placing the fingers in the mouth or on the lips (Bucher, 1968; Horan, Hoffman, and Macri, 1974).

Since the act of nailbiting involves a sequence of motor responses and since it appears to have a learning base, it seems reasonable to discuss its development within the context of a motor learning framework. The discussion will focus on the three stages of motor learning as proposed by Fitts (1965) and the ways in which the development and persistence of nailbiting may relate specifically to this model.

Fitts' three phases of skill learning are: (a) the cognitive phase, (b) the fixation phase, and (c) the autonomous phase.

The Cognitive Phase

According to Fitts, "cognitive processes are heavily involved early in the learning of most complex skills" (p. 187). The understanding of a task is the initial learning point in the acquisition of a skill. Sage (1977) commented that the three basic aspects of Fitts' cognitive phase are:

> (1) The goal of the task, (2) The movements which will bring about accomplishment of the goal, and (3) The "strategy" which will work best to produce the desired movements. It may be seen, then, that the learning of a skill does not begin when actual practice starts but before with a cognitive understanding of the motor task. [pp. 364-365]

Sage went on to say that:

> The learner must construct an executive program, or cognitive map, for task accomplishment, based upon the goal. The notion that motor learning involves the formation of some cognitive plan or map has been proposed by several learning theorists. Tolman (1948) proposed the formation of cognitive maps while Miller and his colleagues (1960) used the word "plans" to refer to this initial cognitive structuring. [p. 365]

A molar-level description of the approximate equivalents of the goal, the movements, and the strategy for the nailbiting response would, respectively, seem to be: (a) putting the fingers in the mouth and biting the fingernails; (b) the movements involved in raising the hand to the mouth, in making tooth-nail contact, and in actually biting the nails; and (c) the strategy of establishing a preference for particular fingernails because they are either more convenient to bite or they enable the biting to be more easily disguised. If a finger preference were noted, the explanation given would probably be related to random behavior or even a trial-and-error process. Many motor skills are learned in a random or "trial-and-error manner" (Sage, 1977, p. 365), as are many oral habits (Barnett, 1974).

During this early, cognitive phase of learning, the motor pattern is performed "with more or less conscious attention to the details of the execution" (Sage, p. 365). This phase "may be accomplished in a few moments or a few weeks, depending upon such factors as the complexity of the task, prior experience with similar tasks, perceptual abilities, [and] frequency of practice" (Sage, p. 365). The response of biting the fingernails may not be regarded as a complex task because several of the component movements involved in this response have most likely been in the individual's motor repertoire for some time; e.g., the act of putting the hand to the mouth (Solomon, 1955). Many of the actions of nailbiting are similar to those performed during thumb-sucking, which is considered a natural response of the infant. Hence, this "prior experience with similar tasks" (Sage, p. 365) and the relative simplicity of the nailbiting response perhaps are significant in facilitating its development. In other words, the individual may pass rather quickly through the cognitive phase in acquiring the nailbiting response. As Fitts and Posner (1968) stated:

> The early or cognitive stage of learning . . . allows for the selection of an initial repertoire of subroutines . . . from the available ones that have been developed previously. At this stage behavior is truly a patchwork of old habits ready to be put together into new patterns and supplemented by a few new habits. . . . It is usually necessary to attend to cues, events, and responses that later go unnoticed. [p. 12]

Another factor that enhances the rate of learning a motor skill is the way in which information about the skill is communicated to the individual. This may be accomplished by using the visual, auditory, or kinesthetic channels of communication (Lockhart, cited in Sage, 1977, p. 366).

In 1951, Fitts suggested "that early motor learning is primarily under visual control" (cited in Sage, 1977, p. 367). With regard to nailbiting, it may be surmised that an individual visually inspects his fingers for cues that initiate the biting response; e.g., a broken or rough edge or a certain amount of nail growth. Looking at the nail immediately before placing the finger in the mouth would also provide specific information for correctly aligning the nail with the teeth. The importance of the visual channel in the learning of a skill was emphasized in 1951 by Fitts (cited in Sage, 1977): "Vision is the major error-correcting mechanism used by the individual; as errors in performance become smaller, the appropriate "feel" or proprioceptive cues may become more prominent for error correcting" (p. 367).

As discussed earlier, several researchers (Azrin and Nunn, 1977; Hill, 1946; Illingworth, 1964; Kanner, 1972; Langford, 1972) have noted that the visual modeling effect may contribute to the development of the nailbiting mannerism. The visual model provided by friends or members of the family who bite their nails may be internalized into a cognitive plan of action. Making reference to a possible modeling influence for the learning of motor skills, Sage (1977) noted: "Some form of demonstration is the most direct and economical technique of communicating the task to the learner" (p. 366). Further support is given to his statement by Bandura (cited in Sage, 1977) who found that "observational learning studies have demonstrated that visual observation of another's performance facilitates the learning of skills" (p. 366). Landers and Landers (cited in Sage, 1977) reported: "A demonstration model does facilitate and enhance acquisition of behavior responses, particularly in the initial stage" (p. 366).

The auditory model of hearing others talk about their nailbiting behavior may also play a role in the development of nailbiting. This statement could be regarded as an extension of Sage's formulation that "it is possible . . . for many skills to be learned without demonstration, if verbal models are substituted" (p. 366).

The Fixation Phase

The fixation stage of skill learning has been described as "a period during which the movement pattern begins to fuse into a well-coordinated movement pattern. Spatial (correct body segments are employed for best mechanical advantage) and temporal organization becomes 'fixed.' " (Sage, 1977, p. 369). At this stage, it is indeed probable that the nailbiter begins to accurately judge how much of the nail edge can be safely removed before discomfort is experienced. It might also be conjectured that, as an additional refinement in strategy, the nailbiter might perfect the nail's angle of contact with the teeth to facilitate biting. An individual might also learn additional ways of unobtrusively performing the nailbiting response. These refinements of the nailbiting response may be indicative of the fixation of spatial and temporal organization and also of the elimination of extraneous or unnecessary movements.

Referring to the fixation phase, Bahrick, Nobel, and Fitts (cited in Sage, 1977) stated that:

> Proprioceptive feedback becomes increasingly important after extended motor learning and there is less reliance on visual cues as learning of a motor task progresses. . . . Such factors as prior experience with similar skills, complexity of the skill, practice schedules, teaching methods, feedback, and motivation of the learner will determine the length of this phase of skill learning. [p. 370]

It seems reasonable to assume that during the fixation stage, the nailbiter relies less on his visual sense and more on his tactile-kinesthetic sense for inspecting his nails and for detecting nailbiting cues. For example, by moving a fingertip over the nail of another finger, he may locate an irregular edge and subsequently engage in nailbiting behavior in an attempt to remove the roughness.

The Autonomous Phase

Fitts and Posner (1968) briefly described the final or autonomous stage of skill learning: "Component processes become increasingly autonomous, less directly subject to cognitive control, and less subject to interference from other ongoing activities or environmental distractions" (p. 14). Ellis (1978), in describing Fitts' final stage of motor learning, stated: "Performance becomes highly efficient so that it can be executed in more or less automatic fashion" (p. 231). He added that performance "becomes increasingly immune to sources of interference . . . [for example] we continue to talk while driving a car" (p. 232). Perhaps this immunity to interference explains why the chronic nailbiter can carry on with certain activities, e.g., reading a book, while continuing to bite his nails. With regard to the "*automation* of an activity," Fitts (1965) stated that this stage is characterized by a "gradually increasing resistance . . . to interference from other activities that may be performed concurrently" (p. 188). In this respect, it would be predicted that the chronic nailbiter is not bothered by distractions during nailbiting episodes and therefore his performance in nailbiting is not hindered. In relation to a movement pattern becoming automatic, Sage (1977) stated: "As the movement pattern becomes automatic, conscious introspection about the component parts of the pattern during this phase of learning often results in the so-called paralysis from analysis phenomenon" (p. 372). If this statement can be applied to the nailbiting mannerism, one would assume that the nailbiter would be unable to provide, upon questioning, a component analysis of his biting pattern. This so-called paralysis from analysis phenomenon may in fact provide a plausible theoretical background for the awareness training component of many treatment procedures for nailbiting. The essence of awareness training is to increase the nailbiter's awareness of the motoric components of his response; i.e., moving the arm towards the mouth, placing the hand near the mouth, or placing the fingers in the mouth. These movements precede the actual biting response, but because the nailbiting behavior has become so automatic, the chronic nailbiter is often not aware of these initial movements. To prevent the biting response from occurring, he must learn to recognize his secondary habits (Azrin and Nunn, 1977), i.e., the movements that usually precede and hence become part of the nailbiting act. These may be thought of as those responses that initially were attended to, but, as Fitts and Posner (1968, p. 12) stated with regard to motor skills, later go unnoticed. One might say that the nailbiter must again proceed through the early phase of learning, consciously attending to the details of his nailbiting behavior, in order that he become aware of the components of his nailbiting response. The autonomous nature of the biting response of the chronic nailbiter contributes to his unawareness of the situations in which the habit is most likely to occur. He must also direct conscious attention to his nailbiting-prone situations in an attempt to identify them and to enable himself to take preventive measures against biting when in these situations.

Azrin and Nunn (1977) appear to recognize and capitalize on the importance of the visual modality in motor learning, although they did not provide a theoretical rationale for their procedure. In Azrin and Nunn's awareness training program, for example, the nailbiter is required to analyze his nailbiting behavior by performing the response in front of a mirror. Also related to this aspect of the procedure is the same requirement to perform in front of a mirror when practicing the competing responses.

Methods of Treatment

Stephen and Koenig (1970) maintained that while many hypotheses have been formulated concerning the etiology and maintenance of nailbiting, systematic treatment of this habit has rarely been investigated. They regarded nailbiting not only as a significant problem for many young adults, but as a behavior that is conducive to investigation, since it can be "reliably observed and measured" (p. 211).

AVERSIVE METHODS

Nailbiting was considered by Bucher (1968) to be "quite suitable for a behavioral approach" (p. 389). His investigation of the treatment of nailbiting was one of the first to appear in the behavioral therapy journals. The self-punishment procedure employed in his study involved the use of a portable shocking device. Two devices were made available to the subjects, thus allowing them to choose between two shock intensities. They were to select the device that produced "an unpleasant shock they felt was not so strong they could not use it" (Bucher, p. 390).

Each of the 20 unpaid volunteer subjects, seen individually, was instructed to self-administer the shock "following the act of placing a finger in the mouth or on the lips and to discontinue the behavior as soon as it was discovered" (p. 389). They were required to record the frequency of self-administered shocks. In order that the treatment have potential for success, each subject's cooperation in administering shocks to himself was essential. A possible unwanted outcome of this procedure, as recognized by Bucher (1968), was that both the nail-biting behavior and the cooperation required by the subjects to self-administer shock would be suppressed. Bucher's (1968) explanation for the possibility of this occurring was that both preceded the shock. In order to maintain the cooperation of the subjects in administering shock to themselves, Bucher provided positive reinforcement to the subjects for their cooperation in following the procedure. This took the form of encouragement from the therapist as well as from the subject's own "experience of success in treatment" (p. 389).

Since therapist effects were an integral part of the experiment, three control procedures were employed in order to distinguish between the effects of the shock and the influence of the therapist. The following is a summary of these three control procedures (Bucher, 1968):

1. Four subjects were instructed to administer shock to themselves whenever they put the fingers of their right hand in their mouth or on their lips and to make written notes whenever the left hand engaged in this behavior.

2. The subjects in the second control condition were given different instructions for the nailbiting and nail-picking violations. One of the two subjects in this condition made a note of each time that he put a finger in his mouth, and used a rubber band worn around his wrist to self-administer a painful stimulus "if his two hands touched each other to begin [nail-] picking" (p. 390). The second subject in this control condition was required to self-administer shock for each "nailbiting violation" (p. 390) and to note each incident of commencing to pick his nails. Instructions were then reversed. Personal communication with B. D. Bucher provided further information concerning the reversal of instructions: "Reversal refers to reversal of contingencies between behaviors for a single subject (S13). Reversal occurred on Day 5."

3. In the third control condition, the shock was self-administered for each finger-in-mouth incident but was discontinued after 32 days, before nailbiting was completely suppressed. The subject was then asked to make a note of each finger-in-mouth incident.

Bucher found that in the control condition involving different instructions for each hand, nailbiting suppressed "about equally fast for both hands" (p. 391) in three out of the four subjects. These results equally favored faradic shock and note-taking. Three possible explanations were offered by Bucher for these results: "Shock and note-taking may thus have been about equally aversive; or suppression effects may have generalized between hands (for the responses involved in the beginning of the biting act). A third possibility is that motivational and T factors [therapist influences such as encouragement and authority] dominated shock effects" (p. 391).

When different instructions for finger-in-mouth and nail-picking were followed, it was found that the "violation associated with biting was suppressed more easily for these cases" (p. 391), regardless of whether the consequence was shock or note-taking. Another interesting point was noted by Bucher: "Both Ss reported that finger-picking frequently preceded biting, so suppression of picking may have suppressed biting also" (p. 391).

For the subject in the third control procedure, nailbiting returned to a high rate of occurrence approximately 2 weeks after he discontinued the shock. This finding was interpreted by Bucher as supporting "the importance of shock" (p. 391). He questioned his own conclusion, however, on the basis of a possible interaction between motivational factors and self-recording. In Bucher's words: "An interaction between motivational factors and the experimental condition might have occurred, if the S judged note-taking to be an inadequate stimulus" (p. 391).

Of the 20 subjects in the investigation, including the controls, 9 ceased nailbiting from the first day and 4 reported no biting after the fourth day. Bucher attributed his generally favorable results to "a change in attention to the early behavior being punished" (p. 391). He reported that the majority of his subjects indicated that after treatment they were much more aware of the behavior of placing a finger in the mouth or on the lips. Prior to the treatment, they had not become aware of their nailbiting behavior until it had continued for some time on each occasion. Their increased awareness of the early behavior of the nailbiting act may have been the key factor in the success of the treatment. Once aware, the subjects were able to employ their own "self-control techniques" (p. 391). As Bucher stated:

> Stimuli associated with biting onset are apparently not very distinct for most subjects, and later aspects of the behavior are apparently much harder to control. If early stimuli were to be made more discriminable, self-control techniques of suppression might be more successful. Use of shock may serve to provide this discriminability. [p. 392]

Perkins and Perkins (1976) included punishment in their self-control techniques for nailbiting. It was cautiously recommended, however, in conjunction with the guideline "use punishment sparingly and never alone" (p. 16). The description of one of their techniques was preceded by a statement of the disadvantages of punishment which are:

> Punishment does not teach new behaviors; it merely suppresses old ones. . . . Punishment, by virtue of its aversiveness, tends to discourage some individuals from continuing with their program. It may also have the effect of making . . . [the client] anxious or upset about . . . [his] habit. [p. 16]

Perkins and Perkins suggested that the disadvantages can be minimized "by using a mild punisher such as loss of a reward" (p. 16), like sending a check to a charity or political party disfavored by the individual, or withdrawing a favorite activity.

A self-punishment procedure that they believed would be effective was the use of a rubber band to deliver a sharp, painful stimulus. Although the sensation should be painful, it would perhaps not be as anxiety-inducing as, for example, faradic shock. The instructions provided by Perkins and Perkins for this procedure were: "Take a ¼" rubber band and wear it on your wrist and as you become aware of your attempts to bite your fingernails pull the rubber band about 6 inches back and snap yourself hard and painfully" (p. 17).

Three modes of aversion therapy were examined by Vargas and Adesso (1976) in an attempt to determine their relative effectiveness in altering the biting behavior of chronic nailbiters.

1. In the faradic shock condition, subjects were seen individually and required to engage in a 10-minute period of response-contingent shock. After the experimenter established the shock intensity level, each subject underwent treatment in the following manner:

> Each time the experimenter said, "Bite," the subject was required to engage in nailbiting behavior. This consisted of raising the hand that supported the finger electrodes from the lap to the mouth, executing a single nailbiting response, and then immediately returning the hand to the lap. This sequence was repeated once every 5 sec, or a total of 12 times every minute. On 75% of these responses, a shock of approximately 1 sec in duration was delivered upon initial contact of the hand with the mouth. The three non-punished responses within each 1-min interval were randomly interspersed. [Vargas and Adesso, 1976, p. 324]

The shock intensity for each subject was "set slightly above the level the subject reported as barely tolerable" (p. 324). This guideline for adjusting the faradic stimulus shock was suggested in 1962 by Turner and Solomon (cited in Vargas and Adesso, 1976).

2. Negative practice was administered in a group setting, with the treatment proceeding as follows for the subjects in this condition:

> The members of each group sat in a semicircle facing the experimenter, and upon his signal, engaged in nailbiting gnawing behavior for 10 uninterrupted minutes, 1-min per finger. Throughout this period, the experimenter interjected various comments in an attempt to assist subjects in maintaining concentration on the nailbiting response (e.g., "let's go, bite, bite, bite, keep biting"; "harder, harder, keep pressing, don't let up"). All subjects were also asked to engage in 3 min of negative practice each evening. [Vargas and Adesso, 1976, p. 324]

3. The experimenter applied a bitter-tasting substance to the fingernails of each subject in the third condition. These subjects were seen individually and followed the procedure outlined by Vargas and Adesso:

> Subjects were then instructed to gnaw briefly on one or two of their nails to insure that the aversive taste of the substance was experienced. Each member of the group also received his own bottle of *Thum* to apply daily. The importance of having the bitter substance on the nails at all times was continually stressed at the weekly meetings. [p. 324]

Half the subjects in each of the three treatment conditions were instructed to self-monitor their nailbiting behavior during the 3-week treatment period. The control subjects were seen three times on an individual basis and "underwent a simulated fingernail examination" (Vargas and Adesso, 1976, p. 324) at each session. The Malone and Massler (1952) scale for measuring nailbiting severity was used during these mock examinations, but the subjects were not permitted to see their ratings and the experimenter did not comment on their nailbiting.

An increase in nail length was revealed in all three treatment groups, but no significant differences were found among the groups. The study did show, however, that "self-monitoring subjects exhibited significantly greater increases in nail growth than non-self-monitoring subjects" (Vargas and Adesso, 1976, p. 322). This was evident for "both posttreatment and follow-up measures" (p. 325). During the course of treatment, the mean number of responses recorded by self-monitoring subjects showed a significant decrease. Vargas and Adesso specifically pointed out that "the number of responses recorded during the 3rd week of treatment was significantly less than that of the 1st week" (p. 326).

In commenting on the overall treatment effect that occurred in their study, Vargas and Adesso proposed that:

> The reduction in nailbiting exhibited by all three aversive conditioning groups was primarily a function of nonspecific factors that were independent of the aversive procedures administered. It is possible that subjects were capable of controlling their nailbiting to some extent simply by becoming more aware of it through participation in the study. Indeed, all treatment conditions were similar in that they served to focus attention upon nailbiting behavior. [p. 327]

They interpreted "the reactive effect of self-monitoring" (p. 327) as being in accordance with other research findings. Vargas and Adesso found further support for their findings in an explanation offered by Kanfer and Karoly in 1972, whose statements were summarized as follows (Vargas and Adesso, 1976):

> The essence of self-control lies in the discrepancy between self-observation and a "performance promise" (e.g., "I will *not* bite my nails any more") that an individual has made with himself,

> with self-reinforcement operations functioning to rectify this discrepancy. The effect of self-monitoring or observation may be either accelerative or decelerative, depending upon whether or not the behavior in question is seen as violating or complying with the performance promise. [pp. 327-328]

In applying this hypothesis to their own experiment, Vargas and Adesso claimed that:

> In the present experiment, many subjects may have initially made some type of performance promise with themselves to cease biting their nails. However, inadequate or infrequent feedback of undesirable behavior may undermine the entire self-control process despite the existence of such a promise. In the current investigation, the need for continuous response feedback could easily be satisfied by self-monitoring subjects, who were explicitly instructed to monitor their nailbiting. Non-self-monitoring subjects did not actively engage in self-recording procedures, and violations of performance promises were probably far more likely to go undetected. Hence, the undesirable behavior would not be punished on a regular basis, and non-self-monitoring subjects would not be expected to exert as much self-control over their nailbiting. [p. 328]

SELF-CONTROL PROCEDURES

Horan, Hoffman, and Macri (1974) employed self-control techniques to treat chronic adult nailbiters. Although two subjects were employed in a pilot version of the study, this discussion will focus on the data obtained from the two males and two females who participated in the four phases of the actual experiment. These subjects, whose ages ranged from 21 to 25 years, were seen on six occasions during the 7-week treatment period.

The study consisted of four phases. First was a 3-week baseline period during which the subjects were not given any information about the program. Nonspecific relationship factors, such as therapist concern and attention, were present during this time. The second phase involved one week of self-monitoring, during which the subjects recorded "all instances of placing any one of their fingers in the mouth area." Three fingers would receive three tallies (Horan et al.,

p. 307). In addition, the subjects were requested to self-monitor "environmental antecedents" (p. 307) of the target behavior. The third phase of the study was two weeks in duration and required the subjects to self-monitor and punish themselves for occurrences of placing their fingers in their mouths. The aversive stimulus was delivered by painfully snapping the inside of the wrist with a ¼-inch rubber band worn around the wrist. During the fourth phase, subjects were asked to cease self-punishing the target response for one week but to continue to self-monitor any occurrences of "placing their fingers in the mouth area" (p. 308). Because of the self-monitoring procedure in the previous 6 weeks, "the antecedent conditions of the response were clearly established for each subject and a suggestion was made that [he] might engage in an incompatible response such as fist clenching . . . followed by pleasant imagery" (p. 308).

Horan et al. found the treatment to be very effective in reducing chronic nailbiting. The data revealed a 22% increase in the mean nail growth (i.e., .127 inches or 3.23 mm), but the researchers pointed out that this was probably a conservative measure of the actual nail growth during this period because all of the subjects indicated that they trimmed their nails during the last 2 weeks of treatment. Horan et al. reported that the subjects demonstrated "greatly improved cosmetic appearance" (p. 308) and that the number of digits "showing blood and/or cuticle damage decreased from an average of nine to only one" (p. 308). A follow-up evaluation revealed that "none of the subjects' fingers showed any signs of self-inflicted nail or cuticle damage" (p. 308). The daily frequency of the self-recorded response of placing a finger in the mouth, regardless of whether biting ensued, declined from 16 to 2. Horan et al. commented that nonspecific factors such as therapist attention, motivation, volunteering for treatment, and instrument reactivity did not seem to be contributing factors, since improvement was minimal during the baseline period.

In evaluating the effectiveness of each phase of the study, Horan et al. noted that there was improvement during the self-monitoring phase for three of the four subjects. They believed that an extension of the self-monitoring phase would have produced a decrement in improvement. Their prediction is not explained within a theoretical framework, but is based on the data in the McNamara (1972) investigation. Appreciable gains, however, were made by all subjects during the self-monitoring + self-punishment phase of the program, leading the writers to believe "SP to be the essential component of the program" (Horan et al., p. 309). In commenting on the self-monitoring + self-reward technique, Horan et al. reported that "the effectiveness of SM + SR . . . is not clear since all of the subjects trimmed their nails during this phase" (p. 308).

The problem of trimming the nails was attended to in the research by Vargas and Adesso (1976). They instructed their subjects to refrain from filing or clipping their nails during treatment and during the 3 weeks between the posttreatment measurement and follow-up assessment. Immediately after the posttreatment nail length measures were taken at the end of 4 weeks, however, the subjects "were then given the opportunity to trim their fingernails in the presence of the experimenter . . . with the restriction that the length of each nail could not be cut shorter than its pretreatment length" (Vargas and Adesso, p. 324).

McNamara (1972) studied the effectiveness of six different self-monitoring techniques in the treatment of nailbiting. Volunteer male and female college students who participated in the 4-week study were current nailbiters with a long history of nailbiting. The students were assigned to one of six treatment conditions:

> In group 1, Ss were instructed to use a response (finger tapping) incompatible with nailbiting, every time they started to bite their nails, and to self-record finger tapping. Group 2 Ss were like group 1, except that they were not required to self-monitor the incompatible response. Group 3 Ss engaged in the incompatible response but self-recorded the nailbiting response if it occurred. Group 4 Ss were instructed to engage in a resistance response by pulling their hand away from their mouth every time their fingers touched their lips and to self-record this behavior. Group 5 Ss had no active treatment activity programmed and merely had their nails measured at regular intervals. Group 6 Ss were instructed to continue nailbiting and to self-record this response. [McNamara, 1972, p. 193]

Nail length was measured at regular intervals during the study to determine the effectiveness of each treatment condition. McNamara found that the nail length of all groups increased, but differences among groups were not significant. He attributed the similar increment in nail growth in the six different experimental conditions to increased awareness of the nailbiting mannerism among the subjects. Specifically, he suggested that "the Ss were able to control their nailbiting simply by becoming more aware of their problem through their participation in the study" (p. 193).

Recently, Adesso, Vargas, and Siddall (1979) have studied the role of nonspecific awareness factors in self-monitoring treatment procedures for nailbiting. Their investigation dealt with two questions; namely:

> (1) Are the treatment outcomes achieved with self-monitoring alone distinguishable from those produced by nonspecific awareness factors? (2) Can the outcomes produced with self-monitoring alone be enhanced by the addition of incentives to self-monitoring? To answer the first question, the self-monitoring subjects were compared with subjects in two control groups. A "minimal contact" group serve[d] as a control for mere participation, and a "nail measure alone" group controlled for the potentially reactive effects of having one's nails measured regularly. The minimal contact group was expected to achieve results inferior to those of the self-monitoring treatment while the nail measure alone group would achieve comparable results.
>
> An attempt was also made to determine if the effects on nail growth achieved with self-monitoring alone could be enhanced by adding an incentive to self-monitoring. The basic self-monitoring technique was evaluated against two types of incentive conditions for suppression of nail-biting. The three techniques were similar in requiring daily self-monitoring of nail-biting. However, subjects in the self-monitoring alone group were neither rewarded nor punished for changes in nail length over each preceding week of treatment, while individuals in the "positive" and "negative" incentive groups did receive such consequation. The incentive selected was experimental credit, as it was a requirement for satisfactory completion of the course from which subjects were recruited. Hence, while self-monitoring and control subjects were assured of receiving credits for participation, the awarding of credits to subjects in the incentive groups was contingent upon weekly control of their nailbiting. . . Subjects in the positive incentive condition were awarded one credit for increases in nail length over the previous week or forfeited

> the credit for no changes or decreases in nail length. . . . [Negative incentive subjects] were informed at the start of treatment that they possessed four experimental credits. . . . Measurable increases in nail length over the previous week would enable subjects to avoid the loss of a credit, whereas no changes or decreases in nail length resulted in deduction of one experimental credit. . . . Under these circumstances, it was predicted that subjects in both incentive conditions would achieve greater increases in nail growth than those in the self-monitoring alone condition. [pp. 148-150]

Adesso et al. found that:

> Although the self-monitoring plus regular nail-measurement . . . [procedure] does seem to be effective for increasing awareness of nail-biting behavior and for bringing about some reduction in nail-biting, it does not seem adequate for total suppression of the behavior. [p. 154]

The results showed that "subjects in both the minimal contact and nail measure alone control groups achieved the smallest increases in nail growth. . . . Increases attained by the subjects in the nail measure alone group were not different from those of subjects in the self-monitoring conditions" (p. 153). It was also found that the mean nail length of the "minimal contact group differed significantly from the self-monitoring . . . and positive incentive . . . groups and differed marginally from the negative incentive group" (p. 151). The mean nail lengths for all five groups are depicted in Table 23.

Analysis of the results led Adesso et al. to conclude that "regular attendance at scheduled nail-measuring sessions played a significant role in the effectiveness of the self-monitoring treatment beyond mere participation" in the study (p. 153). At the same time, they asserted that it would be erroneous to claim that:

> The increases in nail length experienced by self-monitoring subjects were due entirely to a commitment to attend nail-measuring sessions. While nail measure alone control subjects did not differ significantly from either the self-monitoring or minimal contact control subjects, the self-monitoring groups did differ from the minimal contact subjects. It seems that there was a relation between the amount of attention to nail-biting that a treatment

Table 23 Mean Nail Lengths for Five Groups Across Treatment Intervals[a]

Treatment	*Prebaseline*	*Baseline*	*Treatment Sessions* 1	2	3	4	*Follow-up*
Self-monitoring	122.6	132.0	139.4	145.2	145.6	149.9	158.3
	22.4	23.8	24.4	26.2	28.2	31.1	31.8
Positive incentive	120.5	129.0	140.1	143.1	143.9	152.1	145.7
	15.5	16.2	14.2	15.5	19.4	21.2	15.1
Negative incentive	106.7	114.0	124.7	131.6	136.9	141.7	158.3[b]
	14.4	16.7	18.3	20.1	24.8	24.2	40.8
Nail measurement alone	108.5	118.6	121.4	126.0	126.5	130.1	148.1[b]
	19.2	20.6	22.1	23.8	25.5	27.1	36.7
Minimal contact	106.2	115.9	—[c]	—[c]	—[c]	107.7	121.7[b]
	23.1	23.1				24.5	15.7

From "The Role of Awareness in Reducing Nail-biting Behavior," by V. J. Adesso, J. M. Vargas, and J. W. Siddall, *Behavior Therapy*, 1979, *10*, 148-154. Copyright by the Association of Advancement of Behavior Therapy and reprinted with permission.

[a]These measurements represent the sum of all 10 fingernails presented to the nearest sixty-fourth of an inch. The first cell entry is the mean; the second is the standard deviation.

[b]N = 8 for all cells except these, where N = 7.

[c]No measurements were taken for this group for these sessions.

> necessitated and increases in nail length achieved through the treatment. Self-monitoring and nail measurement afforded subjects more direct and consistent opportunities to focus attention upon their biting and nail length, whereas the minimal contact treatment provided few such opportunities. [Adesso et al., p. 153]

They found "no differential effectiveness" when comparing "the basic self-monitoring technique to each of the incentive conditions" (p. 153). Adesso et al. believed that this finding might simply indicate that inadequate incentives were employed, but noted that the results for the comparisons between basic self-monitoring and incentive conditions were consistent with those of other workers (e.g., Horan et al., 1974; Stephen and Koenig, 1970).

With respect to the number of biting responses reported, Adesso et al. noted:

> The number of biting responses . . . decreased immediately after the baseline week but did not decrease further during the subsequent weeks of treatment. It is conceivable that self-monitoring produces an initial decrement in biting which must then be followed up with additional procedures such as regularly scheduled nail measurements. [p. 153]

Follow-up data were obtained from 37 of the 40 subjects after 4 months and showed that although the nail measurement alone control group had a marginal increase in nail length since the final treatment session, "none of the groups had decreased in nail length" (Adesso et al., p. 152).

SELF-CONTRACTS

The effect of a threatened loss of money on nailbiting behavior was investigated by Stephen and Koenig (1970). The 18 female and 2 male subjects involved in the 5-week study were volunteer nailbiters ranging in age from 18 to 41 years who replied to an advertisement in the university newspaper. Their nailbiting began in grade school or earlier, 19 subjects reported; 16 of the subjects had made previous unsuccessful attempts to break the habit.

Prior to commencement of the treatment procedures, the subjects completed a personal history form, made a contractual agreement, and had their hands photographed and each fingernail measured with a micrometer. The most important provision of the signed contract was a \$25.00 deposit to the experimenter and agreement to forfeit the deposit if the subject did not meet the experimental criteria designated to his/her group. Subjects were required to report twice weekly to the experimenter for inspection and measurement of their fingernails. Measurement was taken from the "base of the nail to the longest portion of the nail" (p. 211) and was compared each time with the previous inspection. Experimental conditions varied among four groups of subjects:

> Group I received \$2.50 of the original deposit after each inspection as a reward for abstinence. Group II received \$12.50 or one-half of the deposit after passing successfully the five previous inspections and received an equal amount at the successful conclusion of the last five inspections. Group III received the total deposit at the conclusion of the experiment, that is, after 10 inspections. Ss in Group IV served as a control and were instructed at the beginning of the experiment that their deposits would be returned to them at the conclusion of the experiment period regardless of any nail-biting violations. The sole requirement was that they should adhere to the inspection schedule. [Stephen and Koenig, 1970, p. 211]

Table 24 clearly illustrates that all four groups increased their mean fingernail length between premeasures and postmeasures.

Table 24 Average Nail Length as a Function of Treatments in Hundredths of Inches

	Pre-experimental	*Post-experimental*	*Follow-up*
Group I	0.37	0.49	0.45
Group II[a]	0.35	0.48	0.38
Group III	0.41	0.51	0.46
Group IV	0.41	0.52	0.46

From "Habit Modification Through Threatened Loss of Money," by L. S. Stephen and K. P. Koenig, *Behaviour Research and Therapy*, 1970, *8*, 211-212. Copyright by Pergamon Press, Inc. and reprinted with permission.
[a]Group II consisted of 4 Ss while $n = 5$ in all other groups.

According to Stephen and Koenig, this overall treatment effect with no statistically significant differences among groups, is consistent with the findings of Bucher (1968).

At the time of the 3-month follow-up, all groups showed a decreased mean fingernail length. The differences, however, between the pre-experimental and follow-up fingernail lengths were generally significant. Subjects, therefore, were "able to maintain some degree of improvement following termination of the study" (Stephen and Koenig, p. 211). One exception to this general finding was Group II, whose mean nail length at follow-up closely approximated the mean nail length at the pre-experimental phase of the study.

Stephen and Koenig reported that during the experiment, all subjects reported twice weekly for inspections as required and "no S violated the provision against nail-biting, including the control Ss" (p. 211). In view of the superior results obtained by the subjects of the control group (Group IV), Stephen and Koenig concluded that factors other than those that were experimentally varied were responsible for the change in nailbiting behavior. This conclusion is similar to that made by Bucher (personal communication), who stated that "there is a large nonspecific component, and my results may largely reflect this." The focusing of attention on nail length by subjects who have made a commitment to an inspection schedule is a factor that Stephen and Koenig suggested requires more investigation. This factor alone could possibly be the key variable in any change in nailbiting behavior. The importance of experimenter characteristics such as "appearance, age and expressed concern for Ss' success" (p. 212) is also a matter that requires detailed examination in future nailbiting research.

In an N = 1 study by Ross (1974), a 33-year-old female chronic nailbiter contracted to pay money to a disfavored organization, contingent on her inability to control her nailbiting habit. During the course of a 90-day period, fingernail length was measured every 9 days. Two conditions were applied depending on the results of the assessment of nail length. The first condition was that all money would be forfeited to the organization for no increase in nail length from one assessment to another. Second, when a length of 2 inches (total for all 10 fingers) was attained, one of the subject's five 10-dollar money orders would be returned by the experimenter. Every 9 days thereafter, the subject would receive an additional money order, providing that nail length did not regress below the target length. If total nail length fell below 2 inches, all remaining money was to be forfeited to the organization.

Ross found that: (a) nail length increased steadily during the 90-day period; (b) the target nail length was reached in 54 days; and (c) nail length had been maintained at 3- and 6-month follow-ups. The subject reported shortening her nails after treatment to increase their aesthetic qualities and to reduce their interference with her typing activities. Hence, any reduction in nail length was not a consequence of nailbiting.

It is interesting to note that the subject stopped nailbiting almost immediately. This abrupt cessation of nailbiting was not necessary, however, since a gradual reduction in nailbiting could have produced a slight increase in nail length every 9 days, which would have met the conditions of the contract.

In responding to a question in the *British Medical Journal* pertaining to treatment for a 16-year-old female nailbiter, Sasieni (1960) suggested a remedy based on weekly self-contracts. The approach entailed systematically reducing the number of nails designated as being eligible to be bitten. Apparently, the duration of this technique was a minimum of 10 weeks, since the individual was to concentrate each week on making one more fingernail ineligible to be bitten. The specific guidelines may be summarized as follows:

(a) Have the client regularly smooth her nails to remove any rough edges and clip any torn bits of skin or cuticle around the nails;

(b) "Explain . . . that it is impossible to bite a smooth nail, since there is nothing for . . . [the] teeth to get hold of" (p. 1520);

(c) Start by making "a pact with herself to stop biting one nail for one week" and instruct the client "that if the chosen . . . [fingernail] comes anywhere near her mouth she is to take it out"; . . .

(d) "The next week a nail from the other hand should be chosen, and an extra nail should be added each week" (p. 1520) until all 10 fingernails are designated as ineligible to be bitten.

In commenting on this four-step procedure, an unnamed expert suggested that it might be successful if during the course of the therapeutic relationship it was determined "that the underlying cause of the symptom would not be aggravated by the removal of the symptom" (p. 1520).

THE ROLE OF IMAGERY

Daniels (1974) found that covert sensitization was markedly effective in treating chronic nailbiting in a 23-year-old male. Two 1-hour treatments brought about a "complete cessation of the nail biting" and a 6-month follow-up revealed "continued abstinence from nail biting" (p. 91).

In this technique, the client was instructed to imagine himself beginning to bite his nails and then to picture himself feeling very nauseated. A relief procedure was used in combination with covert sensitization. The client was told that after he experienced the nauseated feeling, he was to image that he stops nailbiting and no longer feels nauseated.

The following excerpt from the study by Daniels (1974) clearly depicts in detail how covert sensitization was applied to the treatment of nailbiting behavior:

> The patient was instructed to "imagine driving along the highway accompanied by a friend, your arm resting comfortably on the arm rest. As you proceed down the highway you start to raise your hand toward your mouth. As soon as it begins to elevate you get a nauseous feeling in your stomach and begin to feel very ill." Vivid descriptions of vomiting, messiness, and inconvenience to his passenger were also included. In the relief scene in this context, while he began to elevate his hand toward his mouth the preliminary sensations of nausea were followed by the instruction: "As you begin to feel nauseated you decide that nail biting is ridiculous and unnecessary. You immediately begin to lower your arm and hand and as you do so the feeling of nausea disappears and you feel relaxed, confident, refreshed and in complete control of this unpleasant habit." The entire procedure included alternating aversive and relief scenes for a total of 10 sequences of 20 scenes. Similar alternations were applied to other settings in which nail biting typically occurred, such as sitting in a favorite chair at home, attending a movie and working at his office desk. He was instructed to practice 10 self-administered presentations of the alternating scenes twice each day. [p. 91]

In treating a 23-year-old female for compulsive nailbiting, Paquin (1977) employed covert sensitization therapy. Twelve deviant scenes depicting sequences of events that would terminate with the client biting her fingernails were used. In addition, six noxious scenes based on Evans' Fear Inventory (in Paquin, 1977) were presented to the client. In 10 weeks, the client's daily frequency of nailbiting had decreased significantly and the length of all her nails had increased. At one of the follow-up sessions, 40 weeks after initial contact, average nail lengths reflected "gains of more than 50% over baseline levels" (p. 183). Paquin (1977) felt that these results were impressive in view of the client's lack of motivation for change. This low level of motivation was demonstrated by her absenteeism from appointments during 3 of the 10 weeks, which was not supported by good reason nor by notification to the therapist; also, 6 of the 13 home practice sessions were either ignored or not completed. At the follow-up sessions, however, it was reported that the client showed immense satisfaction with her success and with the appearance of her fingernails. She claimed that this improvement in appearance increased her self-confidence in social situations that had once been anxiety-inducing for her. Despite the client's lack of motivation during treatment, covert sensitization appeared to have been successful in reducing her severe nailbiting.

Perkins and Perkins (1976) described several ways in which imagery can be employed in a self-control treatment of fingernail biting behavior. Three techniques were discussed in detail. "The first kind of image to be discussed is a rewarding image. In order to use this kind of imagery you must first identify some kind of imagined reward that you would like" (Perkins and Perkins, p. 14). Once identified, the positive image was to be used by the nailbiter to reward himself immediately upon resisting any urge to bite his fingernails. This should have the effect of "further strengthen[ing] not biting . . . [his] nails" (p. 14).

The second procedure was less pleasant than the first and was undertaken "[to] strengthen the behavior of resisting nailbiting by stopping the image of an unpleasant event" (Perkins and Perkins, p. 14). This approach consisted of two interrelated aspects. First, the nailbiter was to imagine a "very horrifying situation" (p. 14). Second, he could "escape from this unpleasant situation by stopping the unpleasant thought and very quickly imagining the desired behavior of resisting biting . . . [his] nails" (p. 15).

Perkins and Perkins gave the following brief account of their rationale for this procedure: "The desirable image of resisting nailbiting has been strengthened (rewarded) since it was the image that allowed . . . escape from the horrifying, terrifying experience that you were imagining" (p. 15).

A third type of imagining consisted of replacing "the rewarding aspects of fingernailbiting with . . . [an image] that is very unpleasant" (Perkins and Perkins, p. 15). The nailbiter should first "think about any desirable aspects of fingernailbiting" (p. 15). If the individual felt more relaxed while nailbiting or if he liked the taste of fingernails, for example, it would be important to focus on that aspect of fingernail biting. Additional details were given:

> Start by thinking carefully about all the rewarding, pleasant aspects of fingernailbiting. After having focused on them clearly, you immediately follow that with your particularly unpleasant image. . . . This procedure should be repeated each time you have the urge to bite your nails or catch yourself in the act of beginning to bite your nails. Remember to try to use this form of imagery early in the chain of behavior that leads up to nailbiting. [p. 15]

Perkins and Perkins recommended that nausea be the imagined unpleasant event, but they suggested alternative unpleasant images, such as "snakes [or an] open wound" (p. 15).

"NEGATIVE" METHODS OF TREATMENT

Concern for the nailbiting mannerism is evidenced in (a) the sheer number of commercial remedies that are available to combat the habit, (b) the apparent interest of pharmaceutical firms to produce and market over-the-counter remedies, and (c) the continued manufacturing and marketing of these commercial preparations. The third point suggests that either nailbiters, their associates, or both are concerned enough about the habit to go to the expense of purchasing the remedies and the inconvenience of repeatedly applying them to the fingernails.

A British pharmaceutical firm, F. C. Paton (Southport) Limited, produces a product call Paton's Thum, of which Bitrex and oil of cloves are the main ingredients. The director of this company, S. R. Taylor (personal communication) wrote: "Paton's Thum is widely used by all sections of the community, from infancy through to middle age. Nail biting must be a habit that is common right through life."

With regard to a product called Nilbite, R. B. Crowe, Director of the British firm, Branded Pharmaceuticals Limited, in 1975 asserted that "the product [Nilbite] has been marketed without change in formula since 1948 without any claim being substantiated against it" (personal communication). As a result of more recent correspondence with J. H. Holmes, director of Laboratory Facilities Ltd., the British company that now produces and markets Nilbite, it has been determined that one of the ingredients has since been eliminated, but this in no way affects the efficacy of the product (personal communication). Portions of the information contained in a pamphlet that was issued to the public by Branded Pharmaceuticals Limited, and which are still applicable to the product, are provided:

> NILBITE is not recommended for use on children under five years of age.
>
> NILBITE creates a mild to sharp tingling sensation on the taste buds of the tongue. It is not meant to be unpleasant as a taste but merely to act as a reminder to the child (or adult) that fingers or thumbs are in the mouth.
>
> NILBITE coming into contact with the eyes will produce a definite smarting sensation with copious tears. Whilst it might cause the child to complain the smarting will go off in exactly the same way as with shampoo in the eyes; relief can be hastened by a plentiful application of warm water.
>
> NILBITE being water soluble should be applied every time the child's hands are washed. Ideally an eye should be kept on the child to make sure that the Nilbite is not wiped off before its solvent has dried–even so, minute traces under the finger nails which are not removed by this method will probably effect the desired result.

Another product, Stop Bite, is manufactured by Nutress Laboratories Limited of England (Endermann; Kelly [personal communications]). The description contained in the product profile outlines the intended rationale for the chemical preparation:

> The assistance to help break the habit is to provide a 'reminder' each time the fingers stray subconsciously to the mouth. This 'reminder' is a bitter tasting product called STOP BITE.

> STOP BITE is water soluble giving a bitter taste immediately the nail is in contact with the mouth. The product is painted on the surface of the nail using the brush applicator provided.
>
> The bitter taste comes from the most bitter substance known to man–even more bitter than bitter aloes! In the formula we have built in Sorbitol and protein additives to help condition the nails. STOP BITE is in an unobtrusive bottle easily carried in purse or pocket, for instant application after washing the hands.

Thornton and Ross Limited, another British pharmaceutical firm, "for the prevention of nail-biting and thumb sucking" called Nailbite Lotion (Ellis, personal communication).

The Mentholatum Company of Canada indicated that they had modified the formula for their product Stop 'n Grow. Without giving any specific information concerning the formula, Hengelmann stated: "We have altered our formula slightly by deleting two ingredients which will not alter the 'bitterness' of the product."

A. Savage, Public Relations Execute for Salley Hansen Limited, asserts that their product Nail Biter is distributed in "over 3,000 [of their] retail outlets all over the country [England] as well as distribution through larger branches of F. W. Woolworth, British Home Stores, Westons Chemist, Cooperative Societies and some branches of Boots the Chemist" (Savage, personal communication). The product and directions for its use are described below:

> NAIL BITER is easy to use–just brush on the liquid every morning over the nails and allow a few minutes to dry. You'll find the taste absolutely terrible! So terrible in fact that you just won't want to bite your nails anymore.
>
> Remember that breaking any bad habit needs a lot of will-power so your strength together with NAIL BITER will help your nails grow into the longer, more beautiful nails you have always envied. Remember, too, that nails take at least six months to grow completely, so badly bitten nails will take time to show improvement.

Savage also commented on the reminding value of this company's product:

> None of these products [including Nail Biter] by themselves will stop a person from nail biting completely. The bad taste,

which is a harmless ingredient incorporated into the product, acts as a reminder.

According to J. Wright, Director of the National Pharmaceutical Association, England, "one other product . . . has been introduced to the market since 1975. It is Nailoid Let 'm Grow" (Wright, personal communication).

It is interesting to note that the rationale provided by many of these companies for the effectiveness of their products is that the product acts as a reminder to the nailbiter that his fingers are in his mouth. A statement to this effect is found in many of the advertisement profiles or brochures issued by the various companies.

Sarles and Heisler (1978) noted that applying a bitter-tasting commercial preparation to the fingers may be helpful because it functions as a "reminder for the child" (p. 591). They stated, however, that these bitter-tasting substances are "generally inadequate unless supplemented by consistent positive behavioral reinforcement" (p. 591). In addition, they stressed that the child should have some input in choosing the reinforcement to be used. An objection to the use of bitter-tasting substances in the treatment of nailbiting was raised by Jolly (1976), who claimed that they can be "wiped off, thereby creating a situation in which parental authority can easily be flouted" (p. 463).

With reference to negative methods of treating nailbiting, Bakwin and Bakwin (1972) asserted that "punishments, scolding and restraints are of no value and may . . . lead to other difficulties" (p. 510). Similar views appear to be held by Illingworth (1964) and Isaacs (1952) concerning the futility of negative methods used by parents in attempting to stop a child's nailbiting behavior. Isaacs (1952) maintained: "I have accumulated a good deal of evidence showing the uselessness of negative methods of dealing with nail-biting, whether these take the form of scoldings [or] . . . putting bitter aloes or mustard on the nails" (p. 436). Illingworth (1964) contended that "excessive efforts to stop it [nailbiting] . . . are much more likely to fix the habit and cause its continuation than to stop it" (p. 51). Some children, if reprimanded or scolded for biting their nails, will "remain awake at night in order to practice, in secret . . . [their] nail-biting" (Bakwin and Bakwin, 1972, p. 548).

Maberly (1943) suggested that parents should give encouragement to the nailbiter and that this could best be done by having a frank discussion with the nailbiter about his problem. The guideline, although positive, is too general to be helpful. Maberly (1943) was specific, however, to the extent that he did not recommend "nagging, aloes, or even punishment" (p. 365), because of the assumption that such approaches are not only ineffective but in addition may "make matters worse" (p. 365).

Klackenberg (1971) noted that mothers' reactions to their children's nailbiting even at an early age was mild and involved trying "various means to cure . . . [the child] of it" (p. 70). Up to the age of 5 years, nailbiting behavior received a larger percentage of mild reactions than intense reactions from the mothers; of all the reactions, "92% are classified as mild and 8% as intense" (Klackenberg, 1971, p. 70). No specific examples of mild reactions were provided by Klackenberg but those "classified as intense include frightening corrections" (p. 70). Examples of intense reactions to nailbiting are:

> "Bad for your insides," "germs in your tummy," "ugly hands and nails," "might have to go into hospital," together with the purchase of a bitter-tasting substance (Finger-tip) painted on the nails or a rap on the fingers. [p. 70]

These countermeasures were reported by Klackenberg to have been notably unsuccessful.

Billig (1941) outlined a systematic treatment for fingernail biting that was incorporated into a health education project for pupils in grades 4 to 6. The treatment involved the application of an unpleasant-tasting substance to the children's fingers weekly, for a period of 2 months.

Allport and Allport (cited in Billig, 1941, p. 155) suggested that plotted data from a study that employed negative conditioning would result in a J-curve. Consistent with this view, Billig found that charting the data did indeed result in a J-curve for each class of pupils; i.e., when the quassia solution did effect a cure, its effectiveness was usually found to be evident within the first three to five treatments for each of the six groups of children. The greatest decrease in nailbiting, approximately 30%, occurred after the first treatment. The gradual reduction in the number of children biting their nails with successive treatments is summarized in Table 25. Billig (1941) ac-

Table 25 Number of Individuals Who Continued Fingernail Biting After Treatment with a Gustatory Aversion Stimulus. Treatment: Both Sexes

	Grade 6			*Grade 5*		
Treatments	*A*	*B*	*C*	*A*	*B*	*C*
0	15	18	15	22	27	26
1	7	12	9	14	25	20
2	4	11	8	8	20	10
3	4	8	7	8	11	7
4	4	6	7	8	5	6
5	3	4	7	6	4	6
6	3	4	7	4	4	6
7	3	4	7	4	4	6
8	3	4	7	4	4	6

Adapted from "Finger Nail-biting: Its Incipiency, Incidence, and Amelioration," by A. L. Billig, *Genetic Psychology Monographs*, 1941, *24*, 123-218. Copyright by the Journal Press and reprinted with permission.
A, B, and C refer to the three groups into which the nailbiters in each grade were divided. The basis for the grouping was intelligence as assessed by the 1916 Stanford revision of the Binet-Simon tests. The most intelligent students were in Group A; the least intelligent, in Group C.

counted for the increased ineffectiveness of additional treatments in this way:

> There probably occurs an adaptation to the treatment, rendering it ineffective. It follows, if this procedure is to succeed it will do so within the first few treatments, otherwise it will only tend to stabilize, to a greater extent, this behavior. [p. 159]

No further improvement took place after the fifth treatment. According to Billig (1941), it was possible that some of the pupils experienced a relapse after completing the experiment.

Bakwin and Bakwin (1972) stressed the importance of positive reinforcement for nailbiters during treatment: "Encouragement and praise are important, since it takes weeks for the nails to grow and the child is apt to become impatient and discouraged" (p. 510). Another statement made by Bakwin and Bakwin (1972) was related to the possible reinforcing function of visible nail growth. In their brief discussion of nailbiting behavior, they suggested that: "Sometimes the child may be urged to save one nail, meanwhile biting the others if necessary. When the one nail is long, that may be sufficient incentive for the child to stop biting the nails entirely and to let all grow long" (p. 510). Bakwin and Bakwin recommended gum-chewing as a substitute for nailbiting "in exciting situations, as when watching television or while at the movies" (p. 510).

At least one published medical report (Rushforth, 1951) has questioned the therapeutic value of treating nailbiting by negative methods. Rushforth asserted that the often-prescribed remedies of "painting of the fingers with bitter aloes or quinine, wearing of gloves at bedtime, and even splinting of the hands to make the nails inaccessible" (p. 193) only serve to increase the child's anxiety. This medical authority believed that making the child feel guilty about his nailbiting is "largely caused by the parental disapproval" (p. 193) and would only exacerbate the nailbiting. According to Rushforth: "This guilt may greatly increase the child's difficulty and create a vicious circle of guilt—fear of punishment → more nail biting → more guilt → more fear —a circle not easily broken" (p. 193).

Massler and Malone (1950) stressed that education of the nailbiter's parents is a critical factor in the treatment of nailbiting, since parents should be made aware that "all punitive measures, intentional or otherwise, are to be condemned" (p. 529). Coleman and McCalley (1948a) summarized the views held by a number of researchers, including Wechsler (1931) and Bevans (1945), with respect to the treatment of nailbiting by negative methods:

> Most investigators agree that the symptomatic treatment of nail-biting by restraint, bitter applications, scolding, and threats is of little value. Rather they emphasize tolerance, understanding, and therapy directed toward helping the nail-biter to achieve a more adequate overall personality adjustment. [Coleman and McCalley, 1948a, p. 517]

In commenting on superficial remedies such as "scolding and punishing, bribing and depriving of privileges, and horrible-tasting concoctions painted on [the nails]" (p. 58), Bevans (1945) reported that they all appear to be in vain and listed a number of general suggestions for parents of nailbiting children:

1. Instead of scolding and shaming the nailbiter, use occasional gentle reminders.

2. Do not expect the child to be consistent in his efforts to correct and prevent the habit.

3. Generally ignore the habit and use praise when the child does not exhibit nailbiting.

4. Look for causes of nervousness, such as troubles at school with studies or the teacher.

5. Be sure the child gets plenty of rest, fresh air, activity, and good food. Activity should be balanced between outdoor play and opportunities to use the mind, hands, and emotions in arts, mechanics, and handcraft.

Bevans generally discouraged giving rewards to children for attempting to stop nailbiting unless they provided sufficient incentive to break the habit.

Shahovitch (1945) held views that were similar to those of Bevans. For the child who has just begun to bite his nails, Shahovitch (1945) recommended: "don't scold or shame" the nailbiter; try to "find the cause of his nervousness or worry" (p. 304). This would include monitoring the child's radio programs and movies and discontinuing those during which the child was observed biting his nails. Prevention involved reducing the "nervous stimulation for the child coupled with health-giving employment" (p. 304). Consistent with this suggestion for prevention, Shahovitch (1945) believed that various crafts such as spinning, weaving, and music (p. 304) are soothing and healing to the nervous system and are more valuable to the child than aimless amusement with crayons.

Perhaps the most interesting advice for the treatment of nailbiting behavior was reported in the "Letters, Notes, and Answers" section of the June 27, 1936 issue of the *British Medical Journal* (p. 1332). Advice was sought for treating severe nailbiting in a 7-year-old girl. Bitter aloes applied to the nails and even taping the ends of the fingers had failed to remediate the problem. The following suggestion for remediation given by an unnamed expert might be effective, in spite of the possible Draculalike appearance of the child:

> The patient's dental surgeon should be asked to fix two caps on the upper first permanent molar teeth. These would keep the incisors from meeting and so prevent the child biting her nails. The caps must not be left on or the articulation will be upset. [p. 1332]

TECHNIQUES RELATED TO CARE OF THE NAILS

Salzmann suggested that enhancing the awareness of and appearance of the fingernails in girls may be effective as a remedial strategy. He wrote: "Arousing a new interest in the fingernails such as the application of fingernail polish has been found helpful in girls" (Salzmann, 1974, p. 318). Boys cannot receive the benefit of such a procedure because fashion dictates that boys do not wear polish on their fingernails (Hurlock, 1949, p. 245). For boys, Salzmann recommended that they "be appealed to on the basis of good sportsmanship or reward for effort in sparing the nails of an increasing number of fingers" (p. 318). Another writer (Illingworth, 1964) held a similar view of treatment: "In the case of a girl, an appeal may be made to her vanity by applying nail varnish or paint, and making her feel that she will spoil the appearance of the nails by biting them" (p. 51). Buying a female nailbiter a bottle of colorless nail varnish or paint was considered by Jolly (1976) to be a simple solution to a nailbiting problem. The child would want to demonstrate to her friends that she is permitted to use nail varnish but will probably wait until her nails have grown before doing so. This supposedly would provide her with some incentive for letting her nails grow.

Massler and Malone (1950) described what they called " 'Reminding' Methods of Treatment" (p. 528) for the management of nailbiting. Their approach was basically a sympathetic, nonpunitive one:

> Once willingness and cooperation are won, measures to "remind" the nailbiter are generally effective. One can use nail polish in the female; an "expensive" manicure (by a beautician, not by the parent), is surprisingly effective. A simple bandage to cover the "wounded" fingers is very effective once the boy (and his friends) are made to understand that this is treatment for the injury and not for the nailbiting. [p. 529]

A brief article in *Midnight* (Bentley, 1975) provided an account of a children's clinic for nailbiting, which is operated in conjunction with a manicure business. The technique is reported to involve 1-hour sessions during which the child and the therapist-manicurist talk about the nails and how to care for them. The child is given a manicure and encouraged to learn how to manicure her own nails. This is accomplished through role-playing activities in which the child pretends that she is giving herself a manicure. At the conclusion of the session, the therapist-manicurist extracts a promise from the child to "keep fingernails and teeth entirely separated" (p. 25). Apparently the technique is helpful. According to the clinic director, the children "keep their promises ... [and] you can really tell the difference from one session to the next" (Bentley, 1975, p. 25).

Shahovitch (1945) favored prevention of nailbiting rather than remediation. She recommended that the nailbiter be taught to push back his cuticles, hence substituting one manipulation for another. Bevans (1945) believed that in addition to the comfort gained from well-cared-for nails, encouragement and interest on the part of the child's parents would contribute greatly to the breaking of the habit.

Different advice came from a writer reporting in the July 4, 1936 issue of the *British Medical Journal*. Based on the work of the child psychologist, Dr. Susan Isaacs, the writer recommended the following cure for nailbiting: "Regular and long-continued application of olive oil to the finger-tips night and morning. The softening of the nails and surrounding tissues seems to reduce the unconscious desire to bite the nails" (p. 56).

EFFICACY OF SYMPTOMATIC TREATMENT

Not all clinicians agree that symptomatic treatment is effective for nailbiting. One medical authority, Rushforth (1951), stressed that "it is not possible to treat the nail biting directly" and that attempts to treat the nailbiting response itself may "cause more serious symptoms" (p. 193). An illustration is given of a 7-year-old boy whose onset of migraine coincided with his checking of the nailbiting habit by a "strong-minded mother" (Rushforth, 1951, p. 193).

In their discussion of nailbiting, Massler and Malone (1950) included suggestions for managing mild and severe nailbiting. In the case of mild nailbiting, they believed that treatment was usually not required and that "the child . . . [would] probably transfer to some other activity at a later age" (p. 528). These writers believed that severe nailbiting was symptomatic of "strong internal stresses" (p. 528) and that treatment should not be for nailbiting but for the cause of the biting. They stressed that emphasis should be on "removing the basic emotional factors causing the act" (p. 528).

The effectiveness of symptomatic treatment of nailbiting was investigated by Smith (1957). His negative practice procedures were based on those of Dunlap (1932/1972) but were briefer. In the Dunlap study, each member of a group of college students was instructed to gnaw at his fingernails for two 10-minute periods daily. The subjects had severely bitten fingernails prior to treatment but it was found that "in less than three weeks, the nails had grown out to normal length, and the biting habit was broken in every case" (Dunlap, 1932/1972, p. 217). Although practice was permanently discontinued after this period, Dunlap suggested an alternative to an abrupt cessation of negative practice. He recommended that negative practice be continued with increasingly longer periods of time between practice sessions in order to safeguard against the occurrence of relapses.

Two of Smith's objections to Dunlap's procedure were (1) that 20 minutes a day for three weeks is too much time to expect from the average nailbiter and (2) that too much time spent in negative practice could possibly "fix the habit permanently" (Smith, p. 219).

The subjects for Smith's (1957) study were selected on the basis of their responses on a questionnaire; those indicating indifference to the habit of nailbiting were excluded. Prior to the beginning of the experiment, the fingernails of the experimental and control subjects were examined and rated for degree of severity of nailbiting. Based on the scale devised by Malone and Massler (1952), overall ratings were given and subjects were categorized as having fingernails that were mildly bitten, moderately bitten, or severely bitten. Two experiments, each involving an experimental and control group, were conducted. In Experiment 1, negative practice involved having each of the 33 subjects look into a mirror and imitate his own nailbiting behavior as vividly and as accurately as possible for 30 seconds without actually biting his fingernails. While viewing himself in the mirror, the subject was instructed to think "This is what I am supposed *not* to do" (Smith, p. 221). The duration of the interval between periods of negative practice was 60 minutes. During this interval, the subject was instructed to not exert any effort in refraining from nailbiting and to feel relaxed and unworried if nailbiting did occur. It was explained to the subjects that the effort exerted during the negative practice period, rather than during the time interval between practices, was the important factor in breaking the nailbiting habit. The subjects were instructed to continue the negative practice sessions for an additional 4 days after their nailbiting had ceased and then to gradually reduce the number of practice periods during the following 2 weeks. They were given a mimeographed sheet of instructions, which they retained as "a guide for self-therapy" (Smith, p. 222). The desire to overcome the habit was emphasized, but the subjects were informed that conscientious practice was even more important. The control subjects, each interviewed three times, received no specific instructions during the first and second interviews, but at the third interview they were given the same sheet of instructions as the experimental group so that they could try the negative practice technique if they wished.

In the second experiment, 24 subjects in the experimental group received a brief lecture on coping and expressive symptoms and the possible value of negative practice in controlling expressive symptoms. They then engaged in negative practice for 10 minutes as a group. Each subject was subsequently interviewed and given a set of mimeographed instructions, identical to those of the first experimental group. The control subjects for this group were interviewed only once, at the time of final evaluation for the control group of the first experiment.

Smith (1957) proposed that the results of the symptomatic treatment would differentiate between those whose nailbiting was a coping behavior and those for whom it was a form of expressive behavior. Successful treatment would indicate that the nailbiting was expressive; failure, that it was a coping behavior. The duration of treatment was expected to vary with individuals.

The results of Experiment 1 (Smith, 1957) indicated that a significantly greater percentage of subjects in the experimental group broke the nailbiting habit (<.05), the percentages for experimental and control groups being 33.3% and 6.3%, respectively. The percentage of experimental subjects in the "improved" category was 45.5%; in the control group only 6.3% had improved. This difference was significant at the .001 level. In Experiment 2, there was again a significant difference (<.001) between experimental and control groups for both the "habit broken" and "improved" categories, with the greater percentages in each category favoring the experimental groups (Smith, 1957).

Since there were no significant differences in results between the two experimental groups, nor between the two control groups (Smith, 1957), the data from both experiments were combined. Further statistical analysis of the combined data for the experimental groups revealed that 37% of the subjects broke the nailbiting habit and 12% showed marked improvement. When the combined data for the control groups were analyzed, it was found that only 3% had broken the habit and 7% showed marked improvement. A portion of the results from Smith, 1957, are illustrated in Table 26.

Smith acknowledged several limitations of his study, which may detract from the experimental outcome. First, any possible value provided by the experiment for treatment of nailbiting by means of symptomatic therapy is restricted to college-age individuals. It may even further be limited to those aged 19 to 22 since "subjects in the age range 19 through 22 did better than those who were younger or older" (p. 227). The analysis of the combined data for the 32 experimental subjects aged 19 to 22 years revealed that 69% had improved. Only 24%, however, of the total number of 25 experimental subjects who were either above or below this age range showed improvement. Second, the factor of suggestion in the mimeographed sheet of instructions may have influenced the experimental outcome. The subjects were instructed, for example, that "there is every reason to expect that it will work for you" and "ultimately there will probably be no more relapses" (p. 222). Third, of the 28 subjects who had "improved," three had developed "the habit of picking at their cuticles" (p. 229). One of these three subjects was also biting at his knuckles and picking at his lips. Smith recognized that the development of substitute habits detracts from the efficacy of the treatment.

Another factor which may limit the generalizability of the experiment is that of the 57 experimental subjects, only 6 were females; of these, 2 improved and 4 did not. Hence the results cannot be generalized to include female college-age students. There may be limitations to the generalizability of Smith's findings, but the overall favorable results may perhaps be interpreted as lending support to the hypothesis that nailbiting is a form of expressive rather than coping behavior.

AWARENESS FACTORS IN THE TREATMENT OF NAILBITING

Increasing the nailbiter's awareness of his habit was an integral part of many of the specific procedures outlined by Azrin and Nunn (1977) for the treatment of nailbiting. They asserted that a habit such as nailbiting becomes strongly established because of a lack of

Table 26 Comparison of Results for Subjects in the Negative Practice and Control Groups

Improvement category	*Experiment 1*				*Experiment 2*				*Both experiments*			
	Experimental group		*Control group*		*Experimental group*		*Control group*		*Experimental group*		*Control group*	
	N	*Percent*	*N*	*Percent*	*N*	*Percent*	*N*	*Percent*	*N*	*Percent*	*N*	*Percent*
Habit broken	11	33.3	2	6.3 (<.05)	10	41.7	0	0.0 (<.001)	21	36.8	2	2.7 (<.001)
Marked improvement	4	12.1	0	0.0	3	12.5	5	11.9	7	12.3	5	6.8
Total improved	15	45.5	2	6.3 (<.001)	13	54.2	5	11.9 (<.001)	28	49.1	7	9.5 (<.001)

Adapted from "Effectiveness of Symptomatic Treatment of Nailbiting in College Students," by M. Smith, *Psychological Newsletter*, 1957, *8*, 219-231. Reprinted with permission.

awareness on the part of the nailbiter, which may be partially accounted for by his unobtrusive methods of biting his nails. They explained that the nailbiting routines adopted by some nailbiters in order to minimize embarrassment are inconspicuous and congruent with some of their everyday activities. The nailbiter, as well as others, may be unaware of his biting because of well-concealed nailbiting activity. Azrin and Nunn (1977) described several activities that may be used by the individual to disguise his nailbiting:

> One of the common concealed forms of nailbiting is to bring your entire hand in front of your mouth with the fingers bent almost into your palm so that an observer cannot see your teeth in contact with your nail. Others are to rest your chin on your hand with one nail in your mouth as if you were in heavy thought, or appearing to be cleaning the space between your teeth with your nail, or appearing to be rubbing your lower lip with your fingers. [pp. 61-62]

Azrin and Nunn (1977) felt that awareness should be developed through: (a) self-observation, (b) role-playing, and (c) concentration on the movements involved in the habit.

Self-observation entails deliberately performing the nailbiting act while the individual views himself in a mirror. This method provides the nailbiter with an opportunity to observe himself and to note movements that occur during the act of nailbiting that he would not ordinarily be able to see. Azrin and Nunn (1977) advised that the individual should make up a list of all the different ways in which he bites his nails.

The second step in awareness training (Azrin and Nunn, 1977) is to describe aloud each part of each method of nailbiting as the behavior is slowly performed in front of a mirror. This is helpful in revealing to the nailbiter that his habit is a complex pattern of responses rather than the simple response he may have thought it to be.

The third strategy, concentrating on the movements that comprise the nailbiting behavior, enables the individual to become sensitive to the initial movements involved in the act of nailbiting and hence to interrupt himself prior to actually biting his fingernails. This training increases the nailbiter's awareness of the frequency and complexity of his habit and enables him "to anticipate and react to each habit movement to eliminate it" (Azrin and Nunn, 1977, p. 61).

Nailbiting awareness is also heightened by instructing the nailbiter to monitor his nailbiting episodes and to assess the magnitude of the problem as determined by the rate of occurrence of nailbiting. This monitoring may provide feedback in the form of reinforcement for continued efforts to stop. Azrin and Nunn (1977) suggested that, for purposes of self-monitoring, the strength of the nailbiting response may be indicated in a number of ways: (a) number of episodes; (b) duration, if the nailbiting mannerism is "a continuing activity, rather than a series of single episodes" (p. 42); (c) rate of occurrence, a measure incorporating both number and time. When a duration measure is used, it is commonly reported as a percentage of the available time during which the nailbiting could have occurred. It could also be used to record the duration of nailbiting occurrences during a nailbiting-prone activity, such as reading. For example, the amount of time spent in nailbiting while reading may be appropriately expressed as a percentage of the total time spent in reading on a given day.

Perkins and Perkins (1976) also included awareness training in their remedial technique for nailbiting. They stressed that the following instructions were important and should be closely adhered to in order to achieve heightened awareness of nailbiting behavior:

> Set aside ten minutes each morning and evening to sit in a quiet place in front of a mirror. Slowly bring your hands to your mouth and go through the motions of biting your nails as though you are really doing it. Say to yourself, "This is what I'm *not* going to do anymore." Concentrate on your arm, hand, and head movements–really observing yourself closely in the mirror. [p. 2]

Table 27 reveals the distribution of self-reported awareness of nailbiting behavior in the studies of Vargas and Adesso (1976) and Adesso, Vargas, and Siddall (1979). For each study, the follow-up percentages pertained to the group of individuals who were still biting their nails.

Vargas and Adesso (1976) reported a significant increase in awareness of the nailbiting response from pretreatment to post-follow-up. They also found that:

> When the pretreatment and post-follow-up awareness percentages were analyzed separately for self-monitoring and non-self-

Table 27 Comparison of Pretreatment and Follow-Up Awareness Percentages for Nailbiters[a]

	Awareness percentage			
	Pretreatment		*Follow-up*	
Awareness characteristic	*1976* *N=61*	*1979* *N=40*	*1976*[b] *N=34*	*1979* *N=28*
Always aware of nailbiring	21.4	15.0	50.0	42.8
Sometimes aware of nailbiting	54.0	57.5	41.2	46.4
Usually aware of nailbiting	24.6	27.5	8.8	10.8

[a]Originates with the author but is based on correspondence with Dr. V. J. Adesso and information reported in "The Role of Awareness in Reducing Nail-biting Behavior" by V. J. Adesso, J. M. Vargas, and J. W. Siddall, *Behavior Therapy*, 1979, *10*, 148-154 and "A Comparison of Aversion Therapies for Nailbiting Behavior" by J. M. Vargas and V. J. Adesso, *Behavior Therapy*, 1976, *7*, 322-329. Copyright by the Association for Advancement of Behavior Therapy and reprinted with permission.
[b]These percentages were determined as a result of a post follow-up survey.

> monitoring subjects, the increased proportion of self-monitoring subjects who now reported that they were always aware of their nailbiting was significant . . . while the corresponding increase for non-self-monitoring subjects was not. [p. 327]

The increased awareness reported by many subjects at follow-up, especially by those who self-monitored their nailbiting behavior, was regarded by Vargas and Adesso (1976) as their most interesting finding. "Such a result provides support for the position that awareness is a crucial factor in the reduction of fingernailbiting" (p. 328) they noted.

In accounting for the increased nailbiting awareness among the subjects in the Vargas and Adesso (1976) study, Adesso et al. (1979) stated:

> Participation in the study may have facilitated control over biting simply by increasing awareness of it. Despite procedural differences in the treatments, each did serve to focus attention upon nail-biting behavior. Second, having subjects committed to regularly scheduled nail-measuring sessions could have inadvertently increased attention to nail length, thereby influencing subsequent biting behavior. [p. 148]

An analysis of pretreatment and follow-up awareness percentages in the 1979 study by Adesso et al. indicated "a marginal increase in awareness of biting" (p. 153). Adesso et al. (1979) stressed that their results must be qualified by two other findings: (a) the mean fingernail length increase from prebaseline to follow-up was a modest gain of .0523 in. (1.33 mm); (b) of the 37 individuals examined at follow-up, 28 "reported biting their nails to some extent . . . [which] is not a very impressive treatment outcome" (p. 154). It is interesting to note that although awareness was generally increased at follow-up in both studies, 28 of the 37 individuals examined at follow-up in the 1979 study reported biting their nails and 34 of the 48 individuals contacted in the 1976 study reported some biting.

SELF-JUDGMENT OF HANDS

An interesting and significant adjunct to a discussion of awareness factors in the treatment of fingernail biting is a study by Wolff (1943). According to Wolff, the hands are mediators for the expression of personality, but few people recognize their expressive value. People generally observe facial expressions and pay little attention to the hands. In Wolff's investigation into the expressive value of the hands, emphasis was on the ability of the subjects to make judgments of their own hands. Photographs were taken of the subjects' hands without their knowledge and were later presented to them, accompanied by the following instructions:

> I will show you some photographs of people's hands. Try to imagine what kind of a person you believe has these hands. Try to describe his personality and write your opinion on this piece of paper. State whether you like or dislike these hands, and also tell the sex of the person. [Wolff, 1943, p. 83]

The same subjects participated in the three phases of the experiment, which are described below:

1. Each subject was presented with three photographs of hands (fingertips downward) on a table in front of him. Two photographs were of the hands of his acquaintances, and the other was a photograph of the subject's own hands. The subject was not told whose hands these photographs depicted. The results for this phase revealed

that none of the 11 subjects recognized either his own hands or those of his acquaintances.

2. In the second part of the experiment, the photographs were presented in a fingertips-upward position and again the subjects were not told that they were looking at photographs of their own hands and the hands of their acquaintances. None of the subjects recognized the hands of his acquaintances and only 2 recognized their own hands.

3. Three days later, the subjects were told that they were to judge photographs of their own hands and those of acquaintances. They were not aware, however, that the photographs were those presented to them in the previous two phases of the experiment. Only one subject was able to recognize his own hands; one other subject recognized the hands of 4 of his acquaintances, but did not recognize his own hands.

Wolff (1943) stated that self-recognition occurred in only 27.3% of the cases in all three phases of the experiment. Because people usually concentrate on the expressive function of the face rather than the hands, Wolff (1943) was not surprised by the fact that "none of the subjects (with the exception of one who said that he was particularly interested in hands) recognized the hands of any of the other subjects" (p. 84). Wolff did find it unusual that very few of the subjects recognized their own hands "in view of the constant opportunities for observing them and the frequent attention given them" (p. 84).

Concerning the three accounts of self-recognition, Wolff (1943) commented:

> Of the 3 cases of self-recognition; one was based not on physiognomical criteria but on an external factor, the unmistakable dissimilarity of the little fingers which the subject recognized. The other two self-recognitions, in the third section of the experiment, give no special hint. Some subjects identified the hands of other people as their own and attributed to them their own traits. We cannot draw any conclusions from the number of self-recognitions and of recognitions of others, for they are both practically zero. [p. 84]

Other external factors that may account for recognizing one's own hands are "the shape of the thumb, the nails, the distribution of the hair . . . [and] scars" (Huntley, cited in Wolff, p. 84). Subjects usually could not recognize their own hands "even if the hands . . . [had] not been photographed but . . . were seen in their natural state" (Wolff, 1943, p. 87). The following excerpt from Wolff's (1943) monograph describes the rationale and procedure for tachistoscopically presenting an individual's own hands to himself for identification:

> In order to meet a possible objection that the artificial manner of observing forms of expression in "copies" might account for non-recognition, we considered the possibility of presenting the subject's own form of expression to him by means of a camera shutter. We used a Kodak 9 x 12 cm., and took the lens away so that the shutter served as a tachistoscope. The subjects looked through the light-opening at the object in the back of the camera during exposures of 1/100, 1/50, and 1/25 of a second. We proved the possibility of perceiving objects in this manner by the fact that the subjects could recognize photographs of acquaintances. They also recognized their own pictures, but only after several presentations and then only hesitatingly. This also held good for handwriting (in the normal position). Then we put an inclined mirror at a short distance behind the camera, hiding it from the subjects. We put their hands in the space between the mirror and the camera, and told them to press two bell buttons there. Thus the hands became visible for the subject in the mirror at the opening of the shutter. [p. 86]

Wolff (1943) found that one factor that contributed to inconsistency of a subject's judgment of his own hands was the manner of presentation; that is, whether the fingernails were presented upward or downward. In one example, he found that:

> The self-judgment on the hand with fingertips upward is longer and more detailed than that on the hand with fingertips downward. Presentation in the more familiar position may explain why the hands appear more attractive and active, more free and flexible to this subject. [p. 86]

The mean number of words used in the self-judgments of the fingers in the upward position was 29.0 as compared to 24.0 in the downward position. This difference did not occur in the judgments of the hands of others.

AZRIN AND NUNN'S HABIT REVERSAL METHOD

The habit reversal method of treating nailbiting has many components; namely, awareness training,* relaxation training, identifying habit-prone situations, identifying habit-associated movements, self-appraisal of habit annoyances, learning competing reactions, rehearsing how to control the habit, getting social support from friends, displaying improvement to friends, and self-recording the daily frequency of nailbiting.

Competing Reactions

According to Azrin and Nunn (1977), many nailbiters have unsuccessfully attempted to control their habit by physical restraints such as sitting on their hands. This type of activity is not, however, an effective means of controlling the nailbiting habit because it attracts the attention of others and prevents the person from engaging in his normal activities. It does not, therefore, meet two of Azrin and Nunn's (1977) four criteria for a successful competing reaction: (a) a competing reaction "should not interfere with . . . normal activities" and (b) it "should be capable of being performed for several minutes without seeming unusual to someone who is watching" (p. 80). The other two criteria established by Azrin and Nunn for a successful competing reaction are: (c) that the activity be incompatible with the nailbiting behavior, and (d) that it increase the individual's awareness of the absence of the nailbiting habit while it is being performed.

From the point of view of Azrin and Nunn (1977), the principal competing reactions for nailbiting are the grasping reaction and the clenching reaction. The grasping response involves firmly grasping a convenient object, while the clenching response involves tightly closing the hand to make a fist. Specific instructions were provided for the grasping response:

---

*For more details about the role and importance of awareness training in the Azrin and Nunn habit reversal method, the reader is referred to the discussion of "Awareness Factors in the Treatment of Nailbiting" (pp. 143-151).

1. Immediately upon becoming aware of the urge to engage in nailbiting or one of the habit-associated movements, grasp an object in a natural way so as not to attract attention.
2. Select objects that would be natural to grasp.
3. Grasp an object which will not interrupt an ongoing activity.
4. Maintain the grasping reaction for 3 minutes.

Azrin and Nunn (1977) asserted that the urge to engage in nailbiting will usually disappear at the end of 3 minutes. They recognized, however, that for some individuals the urge to nailbite might last longer than this and also that nailbiting might even interrupt or occur during the competing reaction. Specific suggestions were given for handling these situations: (a) if the urge to bite has not disappeared by the end of 3 minutes, continue the competing reaction until the urge subsides; (b) if the nailbiting somehow occurs during the 3-minute grasping period, the competing reaction is performed for another 3 minutes. In addition, Azrin and Nunn (1977) offered two suggestions with relation to the 3-minute criterion. First, the competing reaction should be actually timed only on a few practice exercises in the initial stages of treatment to obtain experience in estimating the 3-minute duration of the competing reaction. Second, avoid looking at a clock or watch when timing the competing reaction, because this could be distracting and may interfere with one's other activities.

A number of detailed suggestions for performing the competing grasping reaction in a variety of situations have been offered by Azrin and Nunn (1977)*:

Situation	*Competing Grasping Reaction*
1. Reading a book, magazine, or paper.	1. Hold each half of book firmly with both hands.
2. Writing on paper.	2. Hold pen or pencil tightly with writing hand while pressing on top of the paper with all five fingers of your other hand.

*From *Habit control in a day*, by N. H. Azrin and R. G. Nunn. New York: Simon and Schuster, 1977. Copyright by Simon and Schuster, Inc. Reprinted with permission.

3. Driving a car.	3. Put both hands on steering wheel and grasp firmly.
4. Speaking on phone.	4. Grasp receiver firmly with fingers of one hand while grasping another nearby object with the other hand, such as a pen, desk, telephone mouthpiece, etc.
5. Watching television.	5. Grasp armrests (if any) of chair or sofa; or rest hands on thighs, pressing gently; or if eating or drinking, grasp the food or food container.
6. Talking to someone.	6. Grasp some part of your clothing such as your purse or belt or jacket pocket. If seated, perhaps grasp your knees or thighs.
7. Listening to a lecture in a class.	7. Grasp the armrests, the top edge of the desk, or a pen, or press on your note paper.
8. Riding as a passenger in a car.	8. Grasp the armrest on a door or grasp your thighs.
9. Eating.	9. Grasp the appropriate utensil, or the edge of the tabletop, of the chair armrest, or press on the table. [pp. 84-86]

To facilitate the learning of the competing reaction so that it can be performed in an unobtrusive manner, Azrin and Nunn (1977) recommended that the individual practice the reaction in front of a mirror.

Azrin and Nunn (1977) recognized that at times it may be either very conspicuous or inconvenient to grasp an object. In these situations, such as when walking, or entering a room, the competing clenching response would be a suitable alternative to the grasping reaction. The details of the clenching reaction have been carefully set forth (Azrin and Nunn, 1977):

> When clenching, fold your fingers so that your fingertips are pressing gently against the palm of your hand. Your thumb should be on the inside, pressing gently against your palm. In this position you maintain awareness of the position of your fingertips and your thumb. [p. 87]

Azrin and Nunn (1977) emphasized that it was important to engage in the appropriate competing reaction with both hands and not with just the one that the individual has the urge to bite. There may be situations in which it would be more convenient, however, to perform the grasping reaction with one hand and the clenching response with the other. An example of such a situation would be pressing against a glass that is being held in one hand and clenching the free hand into a fist.

It may be recalled that Azrin and Nunn (1977) believed nailbiting to be often precipitated by rough nail edges and cuticles. Consistent with this view was their recommendation that an emery board be routinely used to smooth the edges of the fingernails and that the cuticles and skin around the nails be regularly manicured. This guideline may help to prevent the mannerism from occurring.

The competing response procedure was of limited value in treating nailbiting, as determined in an early study by Azrin and Nunn (1973). This was illustrated by the finding that all four of the subjects in the study reported relapses. One of the objectives in a subsequent study (Nunn and Azrin, 1976) was to further develop the procedure "so that nail-biting would be eliminated without relapses" (p. 65). The results were considerably more favorable, suggesting that there is an advantage to be gained from the competing response nailbiting treatment. The investigators found that: "on the first day after treatment, the clients' nail-biting was reduced by 90%; and by the end of the first week was virtually eliminated (99% reduction)" (p. 66). Nailbiting severity was measured by recording the daily frequency of its occurrence. In addition, Nunn and Azrin (1976) reported that "nailbiting was eliminated for all clients 1 month after treatment" (p. 66). They also noted:

> Evidence that the mere passage of time did not cause the elimination is shown by the stability of the two baseline measures for the clients in the wait-listed group. . . .

> Evidence that the decrease was not attributable to some unique aspect of the counselors is furnished by the similarity of results obtained by both counselors. . . .
>
> The present procedure . . . was equally effective for a large number of clients, for the severe nail-biters as well as the moderate nail-biters, for the young as well as the old, and for the males as well as the females. . . .
>
> No new symptoms [substitute habits] appeared following treatment. [pp. 66-67]

In explaining why the competing activity was unlikely to develop into a substitute symptom, Azrin and Nunn (1977) proposed that "nail-biting was eliminated so quickly that the client only received infrequent practice using the competing activity" (p. 67). Perkins and Perkins (1976) have similarly recommended engaging in a "competing activity" (p. 8) whenever the inclination arises to bite the nails. According to them, the competing reaction should be enjoyable (e.g., shuffling cards), so that the nailbiter feels "rewarded by doing it" (p. 8), thus strengthening the competing response and weakening the nailbiting. In addition, it is suggested by Perkins and Perkins (1976) that the nailbiter should avoid choosing "competing activities that put your hands around your face, since having your hands in the vicinity of your mouth may increase the likelihood of your wanting to bite your nails" (p. 9). Perkins and Perkins recognized that it may be difficult to find an enjoyable competing activity and in such instances they claimed that it may be necessary to select one that is essentially meaningless and, therefore, not intrinsically reinforcing; e.g., making a fist. Since these particular competing reactions are uninteresting, the nailbiter is advised by Perkins and Perkins (1976) to tangibly reward himself for performing them by immediately "taking a sip of coffee . . . [or] chewing a stick of gum" (pp. 8-9), etc. In addition to being reinforcing, chewing candy and gum has the advantage of also functioning as a competing activity itself, since it would be difficult to do this and bite one's fingernails at the same time. Perkins and Perkins also recommended that intangible stimuli be used as rewards. For example, immediately after resisting the urge to bite or catching himself in the act of nailbiting and performing a competing activity, the nailbiter should focus on an image of a rewarding event;

e.g., someone making favorable comments about his fingernails. Another type of reinforcer involves combining a tangible reward with an intangible one after engaging in a competing activity; for example, applying nail polish and imagining how attractive long nails would look. Perkins and Perkins (1976) stressed, through these and other practical illustrations, the importance of positive self-reinforcement for employing a competing response such as fist-clenching. In this respect, their procedure differs from that of Azrin and Nunn (1977) who, in terms of the competing response, primarily emphasized the characteristics of the activity itself.

Managing Habit-Prone Situations

"Nervous habits rarely occur with the same frequency in all situations" (Azrin and Nunn, 1977, p. 73). This statement reflects the rationale for Azrin and Nunn's (1977) treatment procedure for increasing the nailbiter's awareness of his habit-prone situations; i.e., those in which he is most likely to bite his fingernails. In accomplishing this, the nailbiter will also recognize that his nailbiting is not inevitable in all situations, since he will be able to identify those in which nailbiting does not occur. By identifying those situations in which his nailbiting does occur, however, he is able to prepare himself for these specific situations and prevent the occurrence of the nailbiting act. Azrin and Nunn (1977) suggested that fingernail biting was more likely to occur whenever the "hands are unoccupied" and when the "arms or hands are resting on a table, desk, or the armrest of a chair" (p. 75). They predicted, therefore, a higher occurrence of nailbiting behavior among office workers and students who spend long periods sitting at a desk. A list of nailbiting-prone situations was compiled by Azrin and Nunn (1977) with the intent of helping the nailbiter to remember those situations in which he was most likely to perform the habit. For each habit-prone situation, the nailbiter was asked to indicate whether the magnitude of his nailbiting response was best described as "always," "often," "not often," or "not at all" (p. 77). In addition, he was instructed to imagine himself in each of his typical daily situations and in each instance to ask himself the question, "Do I bite my nails in this situation?" (p. 76). If the reply was affirmative, he was to add this situation to his list of nailbiting-prone situations.

Rehearsal of Competing Reactions

Before employing the various competing reactions in real-life situations, Azrin and Nunn (1977) recommended rehearsing them. They listed a number of steps to be followed during the rehearsing of these habit-prone situations and the appropriate habit-prevention responses. Following these guidelines should prepare the individual for preventing his habit from occurring in the actual situation. Nailbiters were given the following instructions:

1. Find a place where it is possible to be alone.

2. Select a habit-prone situation for nailbiting; e.g., reading a book in a comfortable chair, and imagine being in that situation starting to nailbite.

3. Describe aloud the precise details of the situation, including arm and hand positions, and also the sequence of actions involved in performing the appropriate competing response.

4. While continuing to vividly imagine this situation, perform the actions involved in the beginning aspects of the nailbiting response and then proceed immediately to acting out the specific details of the competing reaction.

5. Once confident that this particular habit-prone situation will be under control in the actual situation, rehearse the procedure for another situation, and so on, until all habit-prone situations have been rehearsed.

6. Each habit-prone situation should be rehearsed for about 30 seconds, but only a few seconds should be spent in rehearsing the actual competing reaction. Azrin and Nunn's (1977) guidelines were as follows: "One major exception to reality should be allowed during the rehearsal. Don't maintain the competing reaction for the three-minute duration to be used in actuality. Rather, perform the competing reaction for only a few seconds" (p. 127).

Treatment of Secondary Habits

Azrin and Nunn (1977) suggested that a "primary nervous habit" (p. 49) such as nailbiting occurs in association with many secondary movements, which precede each nailbiting episode. A typical sequence of movements, as stated by Azrin and Nunn (1977), is that an individual may first touch his face in a casual, unconscious manner and then start nibbling at his fingernails. In a sense, the face-touching is part of the nailbiting habit. Azrin and Nunn believed that if face-touching always preceded nailbiting, then the nailbiting could be prevented by eliminating the various face-touching responses. They further contended that the primary habit and secondary habit should be treated simultaneously. If the primary habit of nailbiting were treated without regard for the secondary habit, the persistence of the secondary habit in the absence of nailbiting could give the appearance of symptom substitution. This would not be the case, however, but would merely be the result of not treating the secondary habit. In the words of Azrin and Nunn (1977):

> The failure of previous attempts to eliminate the primary habit may be caused partly by this high frequency of secondary habit movements which surround the primary habit. Even if the primary habit was temporarily inhibited, the continuation of the secondary habits would continually tempt one to follow through and complete the usual sequence by performing the primary habit. [pp. 50-51]

In their treatment program, Azrin and Nunn (1977) included procedures for increasing the nailbiter's awareness of his habit-associated movements. He was provided with a checklist of face-touching movements and was instructed to indicate which actions applied to him. He was further told that he must remind himself to attend closely to any temptation in the future to start any of these habit-associated movements. The following three face-touching movements were among those included in the list (p. 52): rubbing the chin, resting the chin or head on the hand, and cupping the hand over the mouth.

Nail-Picking

Azrin and Nunn (1977) have identified the movements involved in two patterns of nail-picking. These are: (a) "using the thumb to pick at the other fingers of the same hand" and (b) picking "at the fingers and thumb of one hand with the thumb of the other hand" (p. 53). Although some nailbiters rarely pick at their fingernails and some individuals pick but never bite, Azrin and Nunn claimed that, typically, a person usually picks at the nail for a period of time and then begins to bite. According to Azrin and Nunn, nail-picking has its own habit-associated movements. They stated that "picking of the nails is typically preceded by touching the fingers with the thumb, usually in a rubbing motion" (1977, p. 53). The following are some of the habit-associated movements to which nail-pickers were advised to attend:

> Staring at your nails.
> Rubbing the edge of your nail.
> Rubbing a roughened edge of a nail.
> Folding your hands together.
> Rubbing the cuticle.
> Rubbing your fingers against your body or arm.
> Rubbing the thumb against the palm side of a finger.
> Sitting with your hands folded in your lap.
> Scratching yourself with the edge of the nail.
> Rubbing an imaginary, or small, piece of dirt between the thumb and finger. [pp. 53-54]

These nail-picking-associated movements, then, may be the initial movements in the nailbiting chain of responses, since nail-picking usually precedes nailbiting.

Relaxation Exercises

Azrin and Nunn (1977) outlined a three-part process of relaxation exercises to help the nailbiter relax when he is about to bite his nails. Their assumption was that the relaxation exercises will reduce nervousness, which in turn will reduce the urge to bite. These clinicians recognized that nailbiting sometimes occurs while one is relaxed and in these instances it was believed that self-relaxation procedures would not help. However, since "most nailbiters . . . do consider nervousness a major cause of their habit" (p. 70), Azrin and Nunn (1977) felt that relaxation exercises were pertinent to any treatment program for nailbiters. A brief synthesis of the three-part process follows.

First, the nailbiter is advised to alter his breathing pattern from one of shallow, rapid breathing to one in which he inhales and exhales slowly, deeply, and evenly. Inhalation and exhalation times should be approximately equal. It is recommended that the individual count to himself when inhaling and exhaling in order to keep the durations equal. Changing to this more relaxed breathing pattern, similar to that adopted during sleep, is the initial step in achieving a relaxed state.

Second, standing and sitting postures should be relaxed rather than erect and rigid. Azrin and Nunn (1977) made specific recommendations to round the shoulders slightly, letting them slouch forward, and to relax the chest muscles. The seated position is one in which the nailbiter is more apt to bite his nails due to the close proximity of his hands to his mouth. It is while sitting at a desk or in a chair that has armrests, then, that this "relaxed-posture aspect of the self-relaxation procedure should be emphasized" (p. 70). Azrin and Nunn recognized that it may be more difficult to follow the relaxed breathing pattern while reading or writing because of the often-assumed bent-over posture, which cramps the chest and interferes with breathing. The individual's sitting posture should be sufficiently erect so as to allow easy inhalation and exhalation. A rigidly erect posture, however, should be avoided since it may contribute to shallow and rapid breathing.

Self-instruction was the third aspect of the relaxation process. If the individual had bitten his nails or performed one of the habit-associated movements, he was instructed to immediately ask himself whether or not he was nervous. If so, he was to perform the self-relaxation procedure while repeatedly asking himself whether he was standing or sitting comfortably and whether he was breathing slowly and evenly. As the relaxed posture and breathing pattern were assumed, the nailbiter was to tell himself "Relax," or "Slow down" until he started feeling relaxed.

Support from Others

Another idea that merits special attention is Azrin and Nunn's (1977) second route to increasing awareness, not only of nailbiting episodes but also of the advantages or positive consequences associated with eliminating the nailbiting habit. As they pointed out, one of the main reasons for the persistence of fingernail biting behavior is "that other people have accepted it as something that . . . [the nail-biter] could not control and have consequently avoided drawing . . . attention to it" (p. 136). Influenced by this observation, Azrin and Nunn (1977) proposed that a necessary step for the continued control of fingernail biting behavior is the social support of friends and relatives. The expression of positive concern and help from others will encourage the nailbiter to continue his efforts to eliminate the habit.

This social-support approach augments the awareness training portion of the Azrin and Nunn (1977) treatment program and involves encouraging people to help the nailbiter to control his habit instead of trying to conceal it from them (p. 136). The specific details of the procedure are:

(a) The nailbiter should enlist the aid of individuals who would like to help him and with whom he spends a lot of time;

(b) These individuals should be instructed to gently remind the nailbiter to practice his exercises if he unintentionally performs the habit in their presence (e.g., by pointing to the nailbiter's fingernails or staring at his hands as a signal). It is essential, however, that these reminders be withheld for a second or two after the individual begins the nailbiting behavior. This provides the nailbiter with an opportunity to perform the competing reaction without any prompting;

(c) The nailbiter should request his friends to encourage him whenever they notice that fingernail biting is occurring less frequently in habit-prone situations or when the general appearance of his fingernails improves. This enables him to develop self-dependence and self-correction;

(d) Friends who are helping should be told the details of the procedure and be given a progress report by the nailbiter on a regular basis.

There would be times, however, when it would be difficult to obtain help from friends and relatives, such as during the night. Although not part of the Azrin and Nunn treatment program, light mittens could be worn, which according to Bakwin and Bakwin (1972) "may act as a reminder that the nails are not to be bitten" (p. 510). Bakwin and Bakwin (1972) felt that a bitter substance applied to the nails also serves as a reminder to the nailbiter.

Inconvenience Review

Azrin and Nunn's inconvenience review has two purposes: (a) to help the nailbiter realize the different ways in which the habit is causing him distress and is interfering with his happiness; (b) to help the individual eliminate his nailbiting if it is associated with a great number of inconveniences or problems. If the nailbiter assesses his habit as causing very little disturbance, then this self-appraisal of habit annoyances may serve to lessen the individual's concern about his nailbiting. In this instance, there would perhaps be little inclination to desist nailbiting behavior. Azrin and Nunn provided examples of nailbiting-associated inconveniences to help remind the individual of the problems he may have forgotten. Among those cited were (a) efforts to conceal the habit by avoiding situations or activities in which it would be obvious and (b) avoiding people who are or may be critical of his nailbiting.

When the fingernails are in near-normal appearance, the individual has opportunities to enjoy the advantages of having intact fingernails. For example, the once-experienced inconvenience and annoyance of deliberately attempting to conceal the fingernails by folding the fingers "inward into . . . [the] palm" (p. 141) can now be replaced by activities such as resting the hands on the table with palms down and fingers fully extended. Further illustrations are cited below:

Nailbiting-associated Annoyance/Inconvenience	*Positive Consequence/ Advantage of Intact Fingernails*
Example 1	
Difficulty in picking up small objects (e.g., coins)	Coins, etc., can be picked up easily
Example 2	
Avoiding card games	Engaging in card games
Example 3	
Avoiding attention being drawn to fingers by not wearing rings	Rings and jewelry can be worn without ridicule from others

Azrin and Nunn (1977) suggested that self-display of improvement will help the nailbiter to continue the efforts needed to eliminate the habit. The nailbiter should display his nails proudly to others so that he can "begin experiencing the benefits of . . . [his] self-control over nail biting" (p. 141). If the individual waits too long to actively seek out once-avoided people and situations, he will be less motivated to maintain his improvement.

CRITIQUE OF COMPETING-REACTION TECHNIQUE

Ladouceur (1979) attempted to determine if increased awareness of nailbiting behavior was the crucial factor in the Azrin and Nunn treatment program for nailbiting rather than "the emission of an incompatible behavior" (p. 313). In comparing the relative efficacy of the habit reversal and self-monitoring techniques, Ladouceur randomly assigned 50 nailbiters to one of five groups: (a) habit reversal; (b) habit reversal + self-monitoring; (c) self-monitoring; (d) self-monitoring + daily graph; and (e) control group. Photographs of both hands of each subject, including the controls, were taken before treatment and at 6- and 12-week follow-up sessions. Data analysis revealed that "the four experimental groups significantly and equally reduced their maladaptive behavior as compared with the control group" (Ladouceur, 1979, pp. 314-315). No significant differences were found between pretreatment and posttreatment measures for the control group. As Ladouceur explained, the results are supportive of the efficacy of Azrin and Nunn's habit reversal procedure. The finding that all four experimental groups showed a significant reduction in nailbiting behavior, however, cast doubt on the necessity of the competing response/habit reversal aspect of the Azrin and Nunn program. The key factor in the successful treatment of nailbiting behavior, as revealed by Ladouceur's findings, appears to be the effect of increasing the subject's awareness of his nailbiting behavior. Ladouceur (1979) further emphasized this point:

> If behavior therapists would be more aware of the crucial role of increasing the awareness of their clients, the efficacy of their treatments could be significantly increased, especially when the target behavior has become relatively automatic such as it is in the case of many nervous habits. [p. 315]

Delparto, Aleh, Bambusch, and Barclay (1977) used the Azrin and Nunn habit reversal technique in treating three adult chronic nailbiters. Azrin and Nunn's program was followed, with two exceptions. One of these was a longer treatment period and a greater number of meetings between the therapist and the subject—one per week. The other exception was the verbal and written information concerning nail care that was provided to the subjects.

During the first session, the subjects were given the rationale for the program and in the second and third appointments, the Azrin and Nunn strategy was practiced by the subjects. The specific components included "response description, response detection and early warning, situation awareness training . . . habit inconvenience review . . . competing response practice . . . symbolic rehearsal, and the social support procedure" (Delparto et al., 1977, p. 319). The remaining sessions were designated for measurement purposes.

It was found that the three subjects were no longer "abusing their nails" (p. 319) by the fourth session, and by the eighth week had nail length gains that ranged from 33% to 129% of the nail length during the first week. At a 6-month follow-up session, nail length had been maintained at 30%, 70%, and 24%.

Delparto et al. attributed their results to the "long-term efficacy of the habit reversal procedure" (p. 319). It seems, however, that such an interpretation should be made cautiously, because the success may have resulted from other components of the program, for example, the subjects' increased awareness of their nailbiting behavior, rather than from the conglomerate of strategies that comprise the habit reversal procedure.

STATEMENTS MADE BY FORMER NAILBITERS AND NONNAILBITERS

Reasons given by former nailbiters for ceasing nailbiting and by nonnailbiters for not acquiring the habit are included in this discussion of treatment methods, since these statements may provide useful information for planning and evaluating therapeutic measures for nailbiting.

On the basis of survey information from 1,077 college students, Coleman and McCalley (1948a) reported that 22.8% of the males and 35.2% of the females indicated that they were former nailbiters. Coleman and McCalley (1948a) summarized the reasons for stopping given by these former nailbiters:

> (1) Social disapproval, especially among the women students who said that the social disapproval of nailbiting was important to them in the early high-school years. Related to this was the

> opinion that the hands tell much about the person, (2) realization of the social value of long, well-kept nails, (3) fear of being infected by germs from the nails, and (4) imitation of parental care for their hands. [p. 519]

Nonnailbiters comprised 47.8% of the males and 45.6% of the females in the study by Coleman and McCalley (1948a). One of the reasons given by nonnailbiters for their having never bitten their fingernails was that they "never had any inclination to do so" (p. 520). Others reported that they had been deterred from nailbiting because of the bad example set by a nailbiter in their family. Several of the men reported that fear of "chiding and humiliation from their colleagues" prevented them from engaging in the behavior even though they "often wanted to bite their nails" (p. 520). Early training in the care of the nails, including manicures given by the mother, seemed to be an important factor in preventing the nailbiting habit from being acquired.

References

Ackerman, J. L., and Profitt, W. R. Diagnosis and planning treatment in orthodontics. In T. M. Graber and B. F. Swain (Eds.), *Current orthodontic concepts and techniques* (Vol. 1). Philadelphia: Saunders, 1975.

Adesso, V. J., Vargas, J. M., and Siddall, J. W. The role of awareness in reducing nail-biting behavior. *Behavior Therapy*, 1979, *10*, 148-154.

Allport, G. W. *Pattern and growth in personality*. New York: Holt, Rinehart and Winston, 1961. (Originally published, 1937.)

American Psychiatric Association. *Diagnostic and statistical manual of mental disorders* (2nd ed., DSM-II). Washington, D.C.: Author, 1968.

Anthony, E. J. The behavior disorders of childhood. In P. H. Mussen (Ed.), *Carmichael's manual of child psychology* (Vol. 2). New York: Wiley, 1970.

Azrin, N. H., and Nunn, R. G. Habit-reversal: A method of eliminating nervous habits and tics. *Behaviour Research and Therapy*, 1973, *11*, 619-628.

Azrin, N. H., and Nunn, R. G. *Habit control in a day*. New York: Simon and Schuster, 1977.

Babcock, M. J. Methods for measuring fingernail growth rates in nutritional studies. *Journal of Nutrition*, 1955, *55*, 323-336.

Bakwin, H. Nail-biting in twins. *Developmental Medicine and Child Neurology*, 1971, *13*, 304-307.

Bakwin, H., and Bakwin, R. M. *Clinical management of behavior disorders in children* (3rd ed.). Philadelphia: Saunders, 1968.

Bakwin, H., and Bakwin, R. M. *Behavior disorders in children* (4th ed.). Philadelphia: Saunders, 1972.

Ballinger, B. R. The prevalence of nail-biting in normal and abnormal populations. *British Journal of Psychiatry*, 1970, *117*, 445-446.

Barnett, E. M. *Pediatric occlusal therapy*. St. Louis: Mosby, 1974.

Bean, W. B. A note on fingernail growth. *Journal of Investigative Dermatology*, 1953, *20*, 27-31.

Bean, W. B. Nail growth: A twenty-year study. *Archives of Internal Medicine*, 1963, *111*, 476-482.

Bentley, A. Clinic helps kids stop nail-biting. *Midnight*, September, 1975, *22* (13), p. 25.

Bethell, M. F. Restriction and habits in children. *Zeitschrift Kinderpsychiatry*, 1958, *25*, 264-269.

Bevans, G. H. Biting the fingernails. *Woman's Day*, 1945, *18*, pp. 18; 58-59.

Billig, A. L. Finger nail-biting: Its incipiency, incidence, and amelioration. *Genetic Psychology Monographs*, 1941, *24*, 123-218.

Billig, A. L. The consistency of finger-nail biting. *Proceedings of the Pennsylvania Academy of Science*, 1946, *20*, 39-43.

Birch, L. B. The incidence of nail-biting among school children. *British Journal of Educational Psychology*, 1955, *25*, 123-128.

Blair, G. M., Jones, R. S., and Simpson, R. H. *Educational psychology* (4th ed.). New York: Macmillan, 1975.

Bowley, A. H. *The natural development of the child: A guide for parents, teachers, students, and others* (4th ed.). London, England: Livingstone, 1966.

Bucher, B. D. A pocket-portable shock device with application to nailbiting. *Behaviour Research and Therapy*, 1968, *6*, 389-392.

Clarizio, H. F., and McCoy, G. F. *Behavior disorders in children* (2nd ed.). New York: Thomas Y. Crowell, 1976.

Coleman, J. C., and McCalley, J. E. Nail-biting among college students. *Journal of Abnormal and Social Psychology*, 1948, *43*, 517-525. (a)

Coleman, J. C., and McCalley, J. E. Nail biting and mental health: A survey of the literature. *Mental Hygiene*, 1948, *32*, 428-454. (b)

Coleman, J. C., and Seret, C. J. The role of hostility in fingernail biting. *Psychological Service Center Journal*, 1950, *3*, 238-244.

Corn, H., and Marks, M. H. Periodontics: Its relationship to orofacial muscle imbalance. In D. Garlinger (Ed.), *Myofunctional therapy*. Philadelphia: Saunders, 1976.

Daniels, L. K. Rapid extinction of nail biting by covert sensitization: A case study. *Journal of Behavior Therapy and Experimental Psychiatry*, 1974, *5*, 91-92.

Delparto, D. J., Aleh, E., Bambusch, J., and Barclay, L. A. Treatment of fingernail biting by habit reversal. *Journal of Behavior Therapy and Experimental Psychiatry*, 1977, *8*, 319.

Drama of life before birth. *Life*, April 30, 1965, pp. 54-69.

Dunlap, K. *Habits: Their making and unmaking*. New York: Liveright, 1972. (Originally published, 1932.)

Ellis, H. C. *Fundamentals of human learning, memory, and cognition* (2nd ed.). Dubuque, Ia.: Wm. C. Brown, 1978.

Fitts, P. M. Factors in complex skill training. In R. Glaser (Ed.), *Training research and education*. New York: Wiley, 1965.

Fitts, P. M., and Posner, M. I. *Human performance*. Monterey, Ca.: Brooks/Cole, 1968.

Fremont, T. S., Seifert, D. M., and Wilson, J. H. *Informal diagnostic assessment of children*. Springfield, Il.: Charles C Thomas, 1977.

Geiger, A., and Hirschfeld, L. *Minor tooth movement in general practice* (3rd ed.). St. Louis: Mosby, 1974.

Gibson, J. *Psychiatry for nurses* (3rd ed.). London, England: Blackwell, 1971.

Guthrie, E. R. *The psychology of human conflict*. New York: Harper, 1938.

Hill, J. M. Nail biting: Incidence, allied personality traits and military significance. *American Journal of Psychiatry*, 1946, *103*, 185-187.
Holt, L. E., Jr., and McIntosh, R. *Holt's diseases of infancy and childhood* (11th ed.). New York: Appleton-Century, 1940.
Honigman, J. Psychogenic and neurogenic skin diseases. In S. L. Moschella, D. M. Pillsbury, and H. J. Hurley, Jr. (Eds.), *Dermatology* (Vol. 2). Philadelphia: Saunders, 1975.
Horan, J. J., Hoffman, A. M., and Macri, M. Self-control of chronic fingernail biting. *Journal of Behavior Therapy and Experimental Psychiatry*, 1974, *5*, 307-309.
Hurlock, E. B. *Adolescent development*. New York: McGraw-Hill, 1949.
Illingworth, R. S. *The normal school child: His problems, physical and emotional*. London, England: Heinemann Medical Books, 1964.
Isaacs, S. *Social development in young children: A study of beginnings*. London, England: Routledge and Kegan Paul, 1952.
Jenkins, R. L. *Behavior disorders of childhood and adolescence*. Springfield, Il.: Charles C Thomas, 1973.
Jersild, A. T., Telford, C. W., and Sawrey, J. M. *Child psychology* (7th ed.). Englewood Cliffs, N.J.: Prentice-Hall, 1975.
Jolly, H. *Diseases of children* (3rd ed.). London, England: Blackwell, 1976.
Kandil, E. Accurate measurement of nail growth. *International Journal of Dermatology*, 1972, *11*, 54-56.
Kanner, L. *Child psychiatry* (4th ed.). Springfield, Il.: Charles C Thomas, 1972.
Kerr, D. A., Ash, M. M., and Millard, H. D. *Oral diagnosis* (5th ed.). St. Louis: Mosby, 1978.
Klackenberg, G. A prospective longitudinal study of children: Data on psychic health and development up to 8 years of age. *Acta Paediatrica Scandinavica*, 1971, (Suppl.) *224*, 1-239.
Koch, H. L. An analysis of certain forms of so-called "nervous habits" in young children. *Journal of Genetic Psychology*, 1935, *46*, 139-170.
Ladouceur, R. Habit reversal treatment: Learning an incompatible response or increasing the subject's awareness? *Behaviour Research and Therapy*, 1979, *17*, 313-316.
Langford, W. S. Abnormalities of psychologic growth and development. In H. L. Barnett and A. H. Einhorn (Eds.), *Pediatrics* (15th ed.). New York: Appleton-Century-Crofts, 1972.
Lavelle, C. The effect of age on the rate of nail growth. *Journal of Gerontology*, 1968, *23*, 557-559.
Lecky, P. *Self-consistency: A theory of personality*. Hamden, Ct.: Shoe String Press, 1961. (Originally published, 1945.)
Maberly, A. Psychology in general practice: Problems in childhood. *Practitioner*, 1943, *151*, 362-369.
Macfarlane, J. W., Allen, L., and Honzik, M. P. *A developmental study of the behavior problems of normal children between twenty-one months and fourteen years*. Berkeley, Ca.: University of California Press, 1954.
Maddison, D., Day, P., and Leadbeater, B. *Psychiatric nursing* (4th ed.). London, England: Livingstone, 1975.
Malone, A. J., and Massler, M. Index of nailbiting in children. *Journal of Abnormal and Social Psychology*, 1952, *47*, 193-202.
Manhold, J. H., Jr. Psychosomatics in dentistry. In W. R. Cinotti, A. Grieder,

and H. K. Springob (Eds.), *Applied psychology in dentistry* (2nd ed.). St. Louis: Mosby, 1972.

Maslow, A. H. The expressive component of behavior. *Psychological Review*, 1949, *56*, 261-272.

Maslow, A. H. *Motivation and personality* (2nd ed.). New York: Harper and Row, 1970.

Massler, M., and Malone, A. J. Nailbiting–A review. *Journal of Pediatrics*, 1950, *36*, 523-531.

McNamara, J. R. The use of self-monitoring techniques to treat nailbiting. *Behaviour Research and Therapy*, 1972, *10*, 193-194.

Michaels, J. J., and Goodman, S. E. Incidence and intercorrelations of enuresis and other neuropathic traits in so-called normal children. *American Journal of Orthopsychiatry*, 1934, *4*, 79-106.

Mitchell, R. G. *Disease in infancy and childhood* (7th ed.). London, England: Churchill Livingstone, 1973.

Morton, R. Visual assessment of nail growth. *Medical and Biological Illustration*, 1962, *12*, 26-30.

Moyers, R. E. *Handbook of orthodontics for the student and general practitioner* (3rd ed.). Chicago: Year Book Medical Publishers, 1973.

Norton, L. A. Disorders of the nails. In S. L. Moschella, D. M. Pillsbury, and H. J. Hurley, Jr. (Eds.), *Dermatology* (Vol. 2). Philadelphia: Saunders, 1975.

Nunn, R. G. Maladaptive habits and tics. *Psychiatric Clinics of North America*, 1978, *1*, 349-361.

Nunn, R. G., and Azrin, N. H. Eliminating nail-biting by the habit reversal procedure. *Behaviour Research and Therapy*, 1976, *14*, 65-67.

Paquin, M. J. The treatment of a nail-biting compulsion by covert sensitization in a poorly motivated client. *Journal of Behavior Therapy and Experimental Psychiatry*, 1977, *8*, 181-183.

Peck, L. *Child psychology: A dynamic approach*. Boston: Heath, 1953.

Pennington, L. A. The incidence of nail-biting among adults. *American Journal of Psychiatry*, 1945, *102*, 241-244.

Pennington, L. A., and Mearin, R. J. The frequency and significance of a movement mannerism for the military psychiatrist. *American Journal of Psychiatry*, 1944, *100*, 628-632.

Perkins, D. G., and Perkins, F. M. *Nailbiting and cuticlebiting: Kicking the habit*. Richardson, Tx.: Self Control Press, 1976.

Pierce, C. M. Other special symptoms. In A. M. Freedman, H. I. Kaplan, and B. J. Sadock (Eds.), *Comprehensive textbook of psychiatry* (2nd ed.). Baltimore, Md.: Williams and Wilkins, 1975.

Pillsbury, D. M., Shelley, W. B., and Kligman, A. M. *Dermatology*. Philadelphia: Saunders, 1956.

Pringle, M. K. *The needs of children*. London, England: Hutchinson, 1974.

Redl, F., and Wattenberg, W. W. *Mental hygiene in teaching* (2nd ed.). New York: Harcourt, Brace and World, 1959.

Ross, J. A. The use of contingency contracting in controlling adult nailbiting. *Journal of Behavior Therapy and Experimental Psychiatry*, 1974, *5*, 105-106.

Rushforth, W. Nail biting. *Practitioner*, 1951, *166*, 192-194.

Rutter, M. A children's behaviour questionnaire for completion by teachers: Preliminary findings. *Journal of Child Psychology and Psychiatry*, 1967, *8*, 1-11.

Sage, G. H. *Introduction to motor behavior: A neuropsychological approach* (2nd ed.). Reading, Ma.: Addison-Wesley, 1977.

Salzmann, J. A. Diagnosis and treatment in the deciduous dentition. In J. A. Salzmann (Ed.), *Orthodontics in daily practice.* Philadelphia: Lippincott, 1974.

Samman, P. D. The nails. In A. Rook, D. S. Wilkinson, and F. J. G. Ebling (Eds.), *Textbook of dermatology* (2nd ed., Vol. 2). London, England: Blackwell, 1972.

Sarles, R. M., and Heisler, A. B. Self-stimulating behaviors. In R. A. Hoekelman, S. Blatman, P. A. Brunell, S. B. Friedman, and H. M. Seidel (Eds.), *Principles of pediatrics: Health care of the young.* New York: McGraw-Hill, 1978.

Sasieni, D. Nail-biting. *British Medical Journal*, May 14, 1960, p. 1520.

Shahovitch, G. P. Don't scold the nail biter. *Hygeia*, 1945, *23*, 302-304.

Shaw, C. R., and Lucas, A. R. *The psychiatric disorders of childhood* (2nd ed.). New York: Appleton-Century-Crofts, 1970.

Sherbon, F. B. *The child: His origin, development, and care.* New York: McGraw-Hill, 1941.

Sim, J. M., and Finn, S. B. Oral habits in children. In S. B. Finn (Ed.), *Clinical pedodontics* (4th ed.). Philadelphia: Saunders, 1973.

Slater, E., and Roth, M. *Clinical psychiatry* (3rd ed.). London, England: Bailliere, Tindall and Cassell, 1969.

Smith, M. Effectiveness of symptomatic treatment of nailbiting in college students. *Psychological Newsletter*, 1957, *8*, 219-231.

Solomon, J. C. Nail biting and the integrative process. *International Journal of Psycho-analysis*, 1955, *36*, 393-395.

Stephen, L. S., and Koenig, K. P. Habit modification through threatened loss of money. *Behaviour Research and Therapy*, 1970, *8*, 211-212.

Stewart, W. D., Danto, J. L., and Maddin, S. *Synopsis of dermatology* (2nd ed.). St. Louis: Mosby, 1970.

Stone, F. H. *Psychiatry and the paediatrician.* London, England: Butterworths, 1976.

Stott, L. H. *Child development: An individual longitudinal approach.* New York: Holt, Rinehart and Winston, 1967.

Thompson, E. T., and Hayden, A. C. (Eds.). *Standard nomenclature of diseases and operations* (5th ed.). New York: McGraw-Hill, 1961.

Vargas, J. M., and Adesso, V. J. A comparison of aversion therapies for nailbiting behavior. *Behavior Therapy*, 1976, *7*, 322-329.

Viets, L. E. An inquiry into the significance of nail-biting. *Smith College Studies in Social Work*, 1931, *2*, 128-145.

Walker, B. A., and Ziskind, E. Relationship of nailbiting to sociopathy. *Journal of Nervous and Mental Disease*, 1977, *164*, 64-65.

Wechsler, D. The incidence and significance of fingernail biting in children. *Psychoanalytic Review*, 1931, *18*, 201-209.

Why take it out on your nails? *Woman*, February 2, 1974, pp. 50-51.

Wolberg, L. R. *The technique of psychotherapy* (3rd ed.). New York: Grune and Stratton, 1977.

Wolff, W. *The expression of personality.* New York: Harper and Brothers, 1943.

Woodward, R. H., and Mangus, A. R. *Nervous traits among first grade children in Butler county schools.* Hamilton, Oh.: Butler County Mental Hygiene Association, 1949.

World Health Organization. *Manual of the international statistical classification of diseases, injuries, and causes of death* (2 vols.). Geneva: Author, 1967-1969.

World Health Organization. *Manual of the international statistical classification of diseases, injuries, and causes of death* (2 vols.). Geneva: Author, 1977-1978.

Index